# DEPRESSION

Learn How to Overcome Anxiety and Depression

(The Natural Way to Heal Depression and Boost Your Mood)

**Michael Blaney**

Published By Michael Blaney

**Michael Blaney**

All Rights Reserved

*Depression: Learn How to Overcome Anxiety and Depression
(The Natural Way to Heal Depression and Boost Your Mood)*

ISBN 978-1-77485-388-7

Legal & Disclaimer

The information contained in this book is not designed to replace or take the place of any form of medicine or professional medical advice. The information in this book has been provided for educational and entertainment purposes only.

The information contained in this book has been compiled from sources deemed reliable, and it is accurate to the best of the Author's knowledge; however, the Author cannot guarantee its accuracy and validity and cannot be held liable for any errors or omissions. Changes are periodically made to this book. You must consult your doctor or get professional medical advice before using any of the suggested remedies, techniques, or information in this book.

# TABLE OF CONTENTS

# Introduction

This book offers strategies and proven methods to diagnose depression in yourself or someone you care about.

Depression is a serious illness that can sap all of the colors from your life. All the joy, pleasure and excitement you had will soon be gone and replaced by a miserable place of stress, sadness, and anxiety. You'll struggle to get out the door in the morning, then will shuffle along the day like a shambling corpse, before finally falling asleep at night. To worry about what happened the day before. An existence that slowly wears you down and makes you a shadow of the person you once was.

Depression is okay. Millions of people across the globe have been in the same boat. Remember that there's a way out of all this misery, and this book can hopefully assist you in your efforts to remove depression from your life. First, admit you have depression. The book contains a comprehensive list of signs and symptoms that are indicative of depression. Once you've acknowledged that you are suffering from depression, it's time now to take the necessary steps. There is valuable advice in this book on how to fight depression. There are three major options in life: self-care and medication. This book will provide guidance to people who are caring for someone suffering from depression. Finally, you will find some great tips in this book to make you happy today, tomorrow, as well as always.

# Chapter 1: Causes Of Depression

It is difficult to identify the cause of depression as there is usually no single cause. It can be difficult or impossible to pinpoint the root cause of feeling low. That's ok. You should know that the causes of this disorder are different for each person. This means that the best treatment approach might differ for every case. The important thing is to determine what treatment works best for your condition, even if it's not clear what the cause might be.

Some people are more vulnerable to depression than others. It can take time for depression to manifest in some cases. Sometimes depression can develop from serious, unpleasant or life-threatening events. Other times it can be difficult to identify the trigger. However, it is important you know the risk factors. This is a great way to quickly treat the problem and avoid depression. Here are some things that have been shown to be debilitating:

Things in your life that can lead to depression: According to research, you may experience depression if constantly placed in stressful situations. These include abuse of relationships, long periods of unemployment and prolonged stress exposure in work and business. These events are more likely that they will trigger depression than any isolated and recent stressful events. If you are already at high risk of becoming depressed, or because of past bad experiences, stress can trigger depression.

Personality: Individuals with certain personality types are more at risk for depression than others. This is especially true for people with low self-esteem, negativity, and a tendency to worry excessively, as well as those with thin skin and are sensitive to criticism.

Family history: Depression is a risk factor that can be increased in certain people, especially those with a history of depression. Your family history does not guarantee that you will experience depression. Even in cases of high genetic risk, there will be other life events and personal factors that can play a role.

Brain chemicals: Research has shown that depression can be caused by changes in brain chemicals. Although the exact mechanism is still unknown, it has been suggested that these chemicals could change. This problem can be caused by changes to the levels or activities of certain chemicals, including serotonin (norepinephrine), dopamine (norepinephrine) and dopamine (norepinephrine). These chemicals are involved in mood and motivation. They also help to transmit messages within the brain. There is a higher chance of getting depressed if there are changes made to stress hormone levels. These changes should be treated promptly. Commonly, severe depression is associated with changes to brain chemistry. This contrasts with mild or moderate depressive symptoms, which are usually based on events in one's past.

Grave medical conditions: - Depression has been shown to be associated with severe illnesses or pain. This is especially true if the treatment is ongoing or long-term. These can lead to depression directly or indirectly, especially if you're prone anxiety, stress, and worry. Note that you can also experience post-natal depression. If not managed properly, this can lead to more severe depression in women.

Drug abuse and Alcoholism: Those who drink and abuse alcohol are more at risk of developing depression than those who do so. This is especially true when alcohol and drugs become a problem. Because substance abuse and addiction can be a problem, it is crucial to tackle it immediately.

As we have already mentioned, depression is usually caused by a combination a number of factors. This means that it is difficult to pinpoint a single cause. The good news about depression is that there are options. Therapy and medical treatment are common. Understanding the potential triggers that can lead to depression is just one part of the puzzle.

# Chapter 2: Understanding Depression

Let's go to the beginning.

What is Depression?

That may seem like an absurd question. You already know the symptoms of depression. This is why you bought this book.

This perspective shows that the question is not absurd.

To solve a problem, it is important to understand the issue well. That way you will be able to determine which solutions might work. The same is true for depression.

This is the simplest explanation possible:

Depression is a condition that affects your mood, thoughts, and behaviour.

To better understand depression, we need to consider the etymology. Latin word "deprimere," meaning "pressing down," gives rise to the term depression.

If you stop to think about this for a second, you'll see that depression can leave you feeling "pressed down."

Depression can affect your life in many ways. The most common areas are:

The Negative Side Effects of Depression

Depression affects your:

#: Levels in motivation

This is likely the one that you identify with most.

Depression can cause you to stop finding the things you enjoy worthwhile. Everything starts to feel hopeless, empty, or lacking meaning.

A project you were excited about suddenly becomes a huge chore. You might feel less inclined to spend time with friends or with your kids if it becomes too difficult.

The worst thing is when you guilt yourself. You'd be surprised at how many times it took me to resentfully complete a difficult assignment that had passed its deadline. It's one thing that makes you feel like a loser.

#: Types Of Emotions

A better understanding of depression and its negative effects on your health can be helped by the many emotions that are experienced during depressive episodes.

One, once you're in depression, your ability feel positive emotions such joy and excitement disappears. Instead, you get negative emotions.

Even though you're confident and capable of doing well, it is possible to become anxious and unsure. This is what I experience as an author. Despite being an author for many years, when I feel down, I have a hard time writing. I also avoid my laptop for weeks.

Anger, which is mainly directed at yourself for being "weak", can be one of most common emotions during depressive episodes.

Even though you might not express it outwardly you might feel the urge to unfairly attack a friend or stranger when you are provoked. The guilt that comes with it is almost always worse.

Other emotions that can be felt during depression are sadness, anger, grief, shame and jealousy.

#: Thoughts

Also, depression has a profound effect on your ability to think clearly.

The first is your concentration. Depression can cause your concentration to drop to unimaginable lows. You may lose interest due to the negative thoughts and feelings that are occupying you.

Secondly, depression affects your memory.

You may find it difficult to recall important information or details when you are feeling low. When it comes to things that have happened or were said to you in the last few moments, your forgetfulness might be more evident.

Depression can affect your self-perception and outlook on the world. Depression can make you feel down about yourself. You might consider yourself a worthless person and deserving of love, success or anything else in your life.

Even your outlook on the future is bleak. You lose sight of all the positive changes you've made and begin to view your future as "all or none." This makes you miserable.

#: Images of the mind

According to legend, Winston Churchill used his depressive episodes to refer to his "black dog" mental imagery.

You will hear many people saying:

"I was going through dark times."

"I was underneath a dark clouds."

"It marked a turning point in my life."

"It felt almost like I was trapped in a deep, dark hole."

The imagery used in depression describes darkness. When depression strikes, you feel trapped in darkness and cannot find a way out. If you were to write down your depression, you'd choose to use dark colors than light colors. This would represent how you feel.

I find it fascinating when people say things like, "I don't see any light at the other end of this tunnel," because that usually indicates some level of depression.

Light therapy is often considered an effective treatment option for depression due to the fact that depressed people tend to have dark thoughts. It is usually done by exposing the individual's eyes to daylight (or another type of white light).

#: Behaviour

Depression can also have an impact on your behavior.

One reason is that you may lose interest and enjoy other activities, like sex, hanging out with friends and watching movies or playing videogames.

The way you view people can change. You may find yourself in conflict with people or arguing. Sometimes depression can cause low self-esteem which can lead you to withdraw from social situations.

Agitation seems to take control of you and you just can't seem relax. Often, you feel like escaping but can't quite figure out how. It's easy to feel trapped or stuck in your daily life. You feel trapped and stuck in your existence, even if you move with little enthusiasm. Instead, your walk is slow and sluggish, with your head always looking down in defeat. Your posture can accurately reflect how "weighed down" and unhappy you feel.

#: Physiology

Depression can also affect your body's natural functions.

First, the anxiety leading to depression mimics the body's natural stress response. This natural system assists you in dealing with potentially dangerous situations, whether they are real or imagined.

When the stress response becomes active, the brain releases adrenaline. In response, breathing and heart rates increase. Blood pressure rises. Muscles contract in preparation to move. This state should last anywhere from 20 to forty minutes.

It usually lasts for longer in a depressed person. WebMD states, if the fight/flight response is not activated for long enough, it triggers the overproduction of hormones like cortisol. Other vital hormones, like dopamine, serotonin, are left out.

This hormonal imbalance can cause problems in your mood, sleep quality, energy levels and sex drive. If you feel depressed you might lose interest and/or eat less, leading to weight problems.

You now know what depression looks like and the adverse effects it has. Let's examine the kind of people that are most at risk.

## Chapter 3: Live For Education

All of life is taught how important education is. We are taught to learn constantly and to grow. This is true even during the war against depression.

Learning

It might seem strange, but learning can be a reason to live. It can also help with depression. How is this possible? Learning stimulates brain activity, obviously. Consider what could happen if a new hobby was discovered or if you returned to school. While you might not believe it, the cure for Cancer or an affordable water system in underdeveloped countries could be within your reach. Who knows what you may be able to accomplish? You want to find out. You don't always have to read books. You may also be able to learn new hobbies. Learn how to make scarves, blankets, and knit for the homeless. Give your creations away and witness the joy that you bring to others. This simple act will help you to have a positive outlook and give you a point of reference when you feel lost. It will also keep you active and busy so that you don't waste time worrying about nothing. The idle mind is bound to have many unwelcome thoughts. But, as we all know, idle hands are the devil's handy work. It is best to keep the two of you busy, especially with something that will be useful to someone in need.

Teach

Do not suffer alone. Is depression a major part of your life? Do you want depression to have the same effect on others? That's not what I thought. Go out and tell your story. Learn from others how to deal with depression. Get together with others to start a support program, then explain to your loved ones how you can help them. Encourage your loved ones to do the same. Use your personal experiences to help others. Write the words, the ideas, and get people thinking about it. Make your struggle tangible for them.

The Next Generation

Did you also know that doing is one of the best ways for teaching? Children actually learn 90% from their parents about how to behave and what they should do. It only makes sense that you are there to help your children act like grown-ups. Our children are the next global leaders, and we want to make sure they know what they're doing. You have to be patient and take your time. Let them feel your pain. They will also see your downfall. Finally, let them watch you triumph over the ghosts and make you a happier, more fun person. Let them know your courage and perseverance. Do not allow them to see you give up. Don't forget that part about you. This is the best part about it. You get to show your kids both sides of your illness. While they may see you fall so they can identify the symptoms and traits of depression, they will also see you rise from the ashes, shining brightly. They will see the transformation. They will be less likely pick on the lonely and quiet child; they won't become bullies.

# Chapter 4: How To Deal With Workplace Depression

Sitting in silence is not an option for a depressed employee. Do not assume that things will improve by themselves. As with all serious medical conditions, depression must be addressed immediately. It is imperative that you seek professional assistance immediately. Your doctor should be consulted about treatment options, antidepressant medication, and therapy before you approach your employer.

Your condition must be evaluated in order to receive the right treatment. To feel better you will need to coordinate your care with your medical professional and stop engaging in harmful behaviors like smoking and drinking. Although they may offer some temporary relief, such vices as smoking, drinking, or using drugs can make you sick and worsen your condition.

Primary care providers can also help. A referral to a professional in mental health may be possible if you are offered an employee assistance program by your employer. Your identity and condition will be kept confidential by employee assistance programs. It is not necessary to worry about other co-workers finding out.

Proper treatment is crucial, even though this could mean higher premiums. For instance, you may be asked if you want to buy a health insurance plan in the open market. In addition, the National Health Care Act of last year may enable you to receive insurance that covers depression and other mental disorders.

Recognize You Have a Problem

Do not be afraid telling your employer what you are going through. Clare Miller from Partnership for Workplace Mental Health (American Psychiatric Foundation), says that employees should adopt effective mental health strategies. She advises depression sufferers to be mindful of what they wish to accomplish with their revelation.

It can be difficult and time-consuming to disclose your condition. But, this may be necessary in order to receive special accommodations for you job. For example, if you are taking a new medication making you drowsy or if you need to work later in your day, you may need a different start time. If you are feeling unwell, you might have to take a sick vacation.

If you're experiencing depression and it is affecting your work performance in a negative way, your best bet is to tell your boss or human resources. It is important that you do it early so you can avoid getting negative performance evaluations. Most companies also require proof of medical status, so make sure you have the proper documentation.

Consider your work environment. Even though depression isn't as stigmatized as it once was, it still exists. This is why you need to take into account the culture at work. Some companies are more progressive, tolerant than other.

The Americans with Disabilities Act requires employers with at most fifteen employees with serious mental disorders to not discriminate against them and instead offer accommodation to disabled employees. This law protects you, but you must disclose to your employer your medical conditions.

Employers these day are more understanding than ten to 20 years ago. This will make it easier to deal with your depression. Employers understand that good mental well-being is essential for business success. You can't expect your employer will always be there for you. You can still get the support that you need if there is a supportive working environment.

# Chapter 5: Background Information On Depression

It is normal to feel moody, sad, and down from time-to-time. You will find that you feel better once the wounds are closed or when things have changed. We all experience ups and also downs.

American culture tends to view sadness as weakness or failure.

This does not mean we should ignore the suffering of others, nor should we try to ease our own suffering. However, we must accept sadness or depression as natural state of mind. Sometimes, they might be valid responses to certain events. In these cases we should not treat them as weak.

Depression can lead to the same feelings people experience when they feel sad, depressed, or insecure. Depression sufferers experience these same feelings, but they are more intensely felt and for longer periods of the time.

Many people don't feel depressed by sudden bouts of sadness or grief. They experience long periods with low moods that lead to a negative feedback loop. Feelings of sadness can cause feelings of unworthiness and make them feel incapable of making decisions for themselves. This is why it can be so difficult to help someone with depression. Many people struggle to get help or to see the universe in a balanced and hopeful manner that suggests happiness.

It's difficult to comprehend all of the above. Let us start by clarifying some points. First, let's clarify what depression is.

What is Depression?

Depression is a chronic, intense, and lasting state of sadness. Depression is often manifested by severe feelings of depression and despondency. People who suffer from it feel depressed and sad and lose interest in things they once loved.

These feelings are often ongoing and may be a sign of depression. These people feel sad, and it can be difficult to find a positive or happy place. Even pleasurable pursuits are difficult to make them feel much joy.

Depression can cause people get stuck in stressful or critical thoughts. Sometimes, they will go over these thoughts again and again until they become hallucinatory (and sometimes even delusion).

People with depression often experience physical symptoms like fatigue, weight loss or weight gain, mood swings and slow behavior. Sleeplessness can be caused when there is too much stress or sadness.

It can sometimes be hard to determine what we mean when we speak of depression. Many of us have heard people say "I'm feeling a little depressed", but we often interpret that to refer to a temporary state.

Depression is also known as a "mental disorder" or mental illness. When a mental problem is so severe that it is affecting our daily lives, and causing us to have real problems with our relationships and personal lives, depression is called such.

There are many kinds of depression.

It would take a lot of effort to explore all of these types of depression. Bipolar disorder and other disorders are more complex to manage, but we can view them all in terms clinical and situational (or circumstantial), depression.

Situational depression can exhibit many of same symptoms as clinical depressive disorder, but is often caused by an unforeseen event. It could be postpartum, seasonal or even postpartum depressive disorder. However it usually occurs in response to a life-threatening event or extremely dire circumstances.

Situational depression will only be diagnosed if someone has suffered from depression within the last 90 days. This type can be treated by exercise and a short course medication.

Contrary, clinical depression is usually not curable and can almost never be cured on its own. This book will assist you in approaching both types of depressed people, but individuals with situational may not need the same type long term treatment.

Regardless of your type of depression, you can apply similar strategies to address different types. Many of the underlying issues will respond well to similar treatments.

You should keep in mind that everyone is different and each person's way to overcome depression will be different.

It should be obvious that anyone who is suffering from severe depression should seek professional treatment. However, we will later discuss how to do so.

It can be hard to believe that those suffering from depression have less control over their moods. People would love to believe that if someone who is depressed tried harder, had more grit, and took it all in, they would be able to get better.

This is the main problem in caring for someone with depressive disorder. Even though it has symptoms many of us have seen and experienced, it requires deeper and longer-lasting treatment. Even though clinical depression can be managed, it is not something that will disappear.

Being able to empathize with the person suffering from depression is a key step in helping them. You should not view it as, "This person is feeling really sad," but instead consider it the same as someone who has diabetes. Just as you can see that a friend with diabetes might not feel too woozy or have dangerously low levels of blood sugar, you should also consider the negative moods and feelings of someone who is depressed as part a wider condition.

To help you get there, let's examine depression more deeply than just the symptoms.

Depression is a real condition that affects the brain of the person who suffers. One treatment for depression involves increasing monoamine neurotransmitters.

A neurotransmitter is just a type in your brain that helps to transmit signals across different chemical connections. They are basically what tell your brain which chemicals to send through your nervous system, and the rest of your entire body.

These neurotransmitters include dopamine and serotonin. Also known as the happiness hormones. Dopamine can reward the body for certain actions and serotonin helps regulate emotions. It is thought that the brain can't regulate emotions without sufficient levels of these neurotransmitters.

These neurotransmitters and their ability to regulate pain are responsible for the many aches, aches and fatigues experienced daily by depressed people.

If you have ever had alcohol to drink (or if your brain has been affected by it), then you will know what it is like for your central nerve system to become depressed. Alcohol can be a depressant and lowers neurotransmission. Consider how it can cause you to make poor decisions. Depression is an example of this.

It's unclear why some people lack enough of these neurotransmitters. Or whether artificially increasing their levels of serotonin, dopamine, or both can help with depression. However, such medications have been proven to be effective in helping people feel better and function well.

Depression goes far beyond chemical symptoms. Recent MRIs show that long-term depressive symptoms can literally alter the structure and function of your brain.

The brains long-term depressed have seen their hippocampus shrink in size. This is significant because the brain's ability regulate emotions and responds to stimuli through the hippocampus.

It is not clear exactly what the effect of atrophy on your hippocampus will be. However, this is the part of your brain that is most responsible for long-term and short-term memories.

One theory that underlies the whole phenomenon is that the brain shrinks and has less capacity to find reasonable solutions to problems. The mind then turns to a few negative memories whenever it encounters certain stimuli.

No matter the reason for depression or its root cause, MRI scans have shown that long-term sufferers of this condition have brains that look different. Medications can be used to treat depression and help them regulate their emotions.

At the very minimum, you can use it to help understand that a depression isn't someone who is sad. It is actually someone who fails to regulate and manage emotions on a structural or chemical level in their brain.

Can I help a depressed person?

It's possible to feel anxious reading this. After all, depression can be a physical condition. There are several ways you can help.

A recent study on mindfulness meditation revealed that it is possible to reverse the shrinkages in the brain by encouraging positive thinking and slowing down your thoughts. A person's mind can shrink when they are sad. However, by stopping it from shrinking, it can help the mind grow back.

The second is that depression sufferers struggle with managing their emotions and seeing things in a balanced perspective. Helping them to see things more realistically can give them hope and help them find a sense of purpose. They are not incapable of doing this, but they struggle to do it naturally.

There are ways to increase dopamine, which you can help with. Also, lifestyle changes can promote better health that can help manage almost all forms of depression.

Even something as simple a joke can trigger dopamine release. This can allow them to see the humor and help them think positively about the world. If you spend the time to get to to know and understand someone suffering from depression, you can do so much.

Research has shown that 80 per cent of people who seek treatment for depression are able to respond within a month. Many of these 20 percent fail because they haven't received treatment.

Tackling depression

Depression is unfortunately very common in many people, despite how little it's still discussed in the general populace. About one in ten women and one of ten men in the world are affected by it at some time in their lives. Some studies also suggest that estrogen may play a role in depression. These numbers are often not reported, especially by men.

The USA Research estimates that around 12% (and 21%) of all Americans will experience some form of depression in their lifetimes. Depression affects approximately 23 million people in America alone and 350 millions worldwide.

Depression can affect any age and anyone regardless of social status. However, certain people are more likely than others to develop depression. Given the neurodegenerative effects of depression over time, it's not surprising that people between 45-60 are more likely to experience depression.

Also, there is a connection between being disadvantaged (poorer and less educated) as well as depression. This link should be understood to be a trigger and not a cause. Having a degree does not make you more likely become depressed.

A person's history of depression can have a significant impact on their likelihood of developing depression. A study suggests that there is a 25 percent chance that your parent suffers from depression. Other studies have shown a lower likelihood of you developing depression (though some suggest it could be as high as 10 to 15%). This can even apply to adopted children.

This combination of anxiety and diabetes can lead to depression that is more severe. Substance abuse and general health problems can worsen depression. Severe illness is also a factor in depression.

Depression can be caused many things including stress, family history or alcohol abuse, medical conditions, sleep problems, poor eating habits, the environment, and many other factors.

It is important to keep these points in mind. While you don't want your friends to become depressed, when you assess a low emotional state, you can determine if this is clinical depression.

Depression is a serious illness that must be treated.

People don't often take depression seriously. They may not seek treatment or receive a proper diagnosis. Many people think that depression will improve over time.

This leads to a worsening effect on the problems, and the brain can experience more changes as a result. This is why intervention and early treatment is so important, especially in the case of severe depression found in young adults or teenagers.

Many are also skeptical about medical treatments and treatment in general. They might believe they are doing well and that they don't need help. Although this might be true, it is possible that things will continue getting worse without making any changes. At the minimum, you should work towards a higher quality of life.

One of the biggest concerns is that people might be forced to take medication. This medication can cause confusion and make them addicted. It is not the right medication for everyone. Doctors are well aware of this fact, as should you. There are many methods that can be used to treat your condition.

Many people believe that depression can be treated with media. They are afraid, for instance, that if a doctor hears they feel suicidal, they will lock them in a padded cell. Oder they may fear their friends will dismiss them as a weakling and freak.

You'll be surprised at how many people feel depressed, and that medical professionals don't seem like the maniacs you see on movies.

Last but not least, depression can lead some people to adopt unbalanced and destructive thinking patterns, as we've already discussed. If you feel you are worthless and society should not waste their resources, it may be difficult to get treatment. They may fear that they will lose an essential and intimate part of themselves if treatment is not available for their depression.

They are all false. Each person can receive treatment. Your personality, creativity, and ability to function are not affected by any harmful mental disorder.

We all know the meaning of depression. But how can we really tell if someone's depressed?

If you don't have the ability to confirm that a loved is actually depressed, it can be difficult to help them. It is important to decide if you're helping someone who is simply depressed or someone with a more serious condition that might need intensive therapy or medication.

In the next section, we'll look at depression symptoms and how to address them.

# Chapter 6: Anti-Depressants (Ssris). Optional

You can't overcome depression with antidepressants by themselves. Patients who have not made any lifestyle changes other than taking medication suffer high relapse rates. William Marchard, a University of Utah clinical professor of psychiatry, studied the relapse rate of patients who tried to get off medication for a first time. The second and third attempts had relapse rates of 50%, 70%, 90%, and 10% respectively.

When used correctly and informedly, anti-depressants can be a valuable tool in our intervention ladder. They have made a significant difference in my personal recovery. They cut down the recovery process and, more importantly they gave me the support I needed to complete the first steps described in the next chapters. The medication gave me the space to think more clearly and make the necessary adjustments in my life. I don't believe I could have done anything constructive without them. The amount of self-loathing I felt, the pain and despair that I experienced in the depths my depression caused me was simply too much. The SSRIs acted as a crutch. Once I had set the remaining blocks of the intervention structure in place, I stopped taking SSRIs. They are only a tool. We have no control over any connotations, subjectively positive or otherwise, that you might attach to them.

It's fine to choose the natural path of overcoming depression. That is also possible, even though it may take longer and might be more challenging.

If you do decide on SSRIs, please keep in mind that the journey is entirely yours. The only thing doctors can do is help you get through this experience. They have never had to go through it. You will be able to make decisions about dosage levels and timeframes for medication on your own, by listening to what your body tells you.

1.What to Expect of Doctors

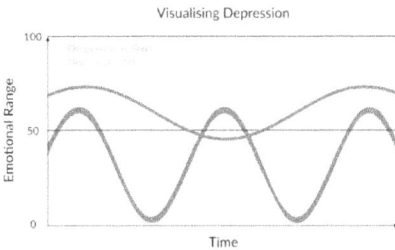

Visualising Depression

"You know what, Doc? I realized that it wasn't working and I left the psychiatrist's office. I had been seeking psychiatric help about a month ago after I moved out of the apartment where my girlfriend of 7 years had lived. I was in a deep depression, felt like I was drowning, and wanted to get help. I didn't know why.

I was thrilled when my psychiatrist diagnosed bipolar disorder in me. The severe pain I felt was known by a name. It was not an uncommon feeling. It could be treated! There was finally some hope. I

41

didn't realize that I was being misdiagnosed. I was in another hole after diligently taking Lamictal bipolar drugs for a month.

My faculties started to be numbened when the medication was administered. My memory was the first to suffer. I would search in another place for the item, only to find that I had lost it. My senses of time were distorted. Then I would find my mind wandering for inordinate periods while reading a book. It would be dark outside before I realized that I was staring at exactly the same page for the previous few hours, but I couldn't remember any of this. Then I noticed the beginnings of speech impairment. I wouldn't have been able to create simple, grammatically-correct sentences in my native languages to communicate with my brother. I was always trying to remember vocabulary and kept repeating sentences three or four times to get them right. After all that brain fog, I realized I'd rather die than lose my last bit of me. That was my capacity to think and reason.

This is in direct contradiction to the fact that the medical field is not equipped or skilled enough to effectively treat mental disorders. I was misdiagnosed based only on what I reported to the doctor and my own self-reporting. I would be in a vegetative state if I had stopped taking the Lamictal medication. My depression would have been confirmed by brain imaging techniques. Unfortunately, this is not a common practice.

My point was not to critique doctors per se. They are capable of doing good work, even though they may have limited training. Depression sufferers should realize that doctors have limited ability to assist them in recovery. My grandfather was a suicide victim, my mother was diagnosed with major-clinical depression, and my brother was diagnosed with the same condition. I found a clinic that provided me with SSRI (Selective Serotonin Reuptake inhibitors) and began self-medicating. I adhered strictly to the prescribed doses (10-20mg daily), but I didn't divulge much to my new doctor. I was content with the fact that she continued to prescribe me the medication.

2.What to Expect from SSRI-Recommended Medication

Antidepressant medication (SSRIs, or Selective Serotonin Reuptake Imhibitors) won't cure depression if used by themselves. That was it. They're not the answer to all your problems. But they can be very beneficial. They were for me. It's important to consider the emotional ranges and spectrum of human beings in order understand their motivations.

Here is my model of how depression can be visualized based on personal experience. A normal, healthy person will experience emotions ranging from 45-70. This means that they experience around 25 emotions (70-45=25). These fluctuations are limited in their range.

These emotions are also averaged at around 60.

In stark contrast, someone with major depression has greater emotional range (amplitude). Our scale measures their emotions from 5 to 55. As such, 50 points are needed to express emotions (55-5=50), twice as many as for a healthy person. Even more important, the average fluctuation of these fluctuations is lower at 30.

The bottom line is that people suffering from depression can feel like they are on a rollercoaster. One can feel relatively well at a reading above 55. For them, this is a high but not a low level. But they then plunge to their lowest point and feel horrible within a matter of minutes. The lows are more frequent than the highs. It is hard to come back above 50.

Antidepressants are beneficial because they accomplish two things. They can reduce the range or amplitudes of emotions. A second effect is to increase the average emotional fluctuation by making emotional lows less prominent. This is because you don't have to fall into the emotional troughs that cause you to feel so depressed and hopeless. These readings are too low and can cause severe depression. I found that SSRIs helped me to recover. Be aware that you can coast and never truly get out of bed if you don't put in the effort. While a reading of 40 might be better than 30, you should still work hard to increase that number.

If you're still not sure whether or not to take antidepressant medication for depression, I would advise you to do so. Although it may take longer, and you may still experience low readings from time to time, the process is achievable. SSRI medication is a useful tool if your case is so complex that you feel like you're losing your way.

Personally, I decided to take Lexapro (active ingredient: escitalopram) since I did not have any one that could constructively support or understand my situation. I was living alone, without work, in a foreign place. My girlfriend of 7 year was dead, and my parents didn't believe I had any depression. What can i say? I really needed the crutch. The SSRIs helped me to reorganize my life and I eventually stopped taking them.

These are some helpful tips for those who wish to pursue the SSRI pathway. These are my accounts and yours may vary.

Timings were important: I found that taking half the dose at breakfast and half the dose at dinner was more beneficial than taking the entire dose in one day. For example, if my Lexapro 10mg/day or 1 tablet/day dose, I would take half and half each morning and evening.

Phases, dosages

Phase 1: Acceleration (1st Month). You may not feel any improvement in your mood during the first 3-4 Weeks. Because SSRIs operate by a specific mechanism, your body must reach a certain threshold saturation. This is a slow process that can only be achieved with low doses. I took half a pill (5mg) every morning for the first seven days to help my body adjust to the drug. Then, I started to take 10mg perday (1 tablet) in week 2.

Phase 2 (Normal dose, duration varies): I continued to take half of the maximum daily dose (20mg), for three months. The medication started working around week 4. My emotional breakdowns were much less frequent, and I didn't cry as often. It was almost like my brain set a limit to the lowest readings I could get.

This period will cause your libido to drop dramatically. I was unable orgasm to be achieved during this period. This could have an impact on your relationship. Viagra is good for men who wish to have sex while taking antidepressants. You can have erections even though it may be more difficult to climax fully with them.

Phase 3 (Duration varies) : At the end of month 5, I increased dosage to maximum 20mg daily. I felt I needed a narrower emotional band to raise the floor. Now I felt well enough, and was able to begin thinking about how I could apply the non-medication techniques to my everyday life. I set out to make my emotional spectrum more like that of a healthy person by bringing it higher on the scale.

Phase 4 (two months): I was most afraid of relapse. I worried that I'd go back to my old ways once I quit taking the medication. I am glad to say that there were two reasons that allowed me not to relapse after the first attempt. First, I had restructured the way I lived so that my emotional profile was comparable to that of an average person. This average reading is much higher than the 40-point SSRI range. Second, the medication was stopped slowly. I stopped taking the full dosage (10mg/day) after the first month. Then I switched to a quarter-of-a-dose (5mg/day) for half the second and third months. Finally, I stopped taking the full dose for every other day. I had some emotional problems in the first month that

I was without SSRIs. I had my brain retrain how to regulate my emotions. But I managed to overcome them.

# Chapter 7: 5 Steps to Handle

# Difficult People at work

Your goal is to meet friendly and cooperative people as you start your new job. It's not always like that. You end up keeping your cool and meeting bizarre people, all for the two-weekly check.

Some people don't like the idea of others being happy. These office colleagues can be difficult to deal with.

It is better to understand them than to try to figure out how to deal.

The Stars

Who they're: The "stars" are the best employees an organization could ever have. They are inspiring and versatile. Their performance supports them, so they are not necessarily bullies. They will not take part in discussions as they believe they are capable. Stars are very insecure and often need ego-stroking.

How to deal. Accept the Stars as they are and let the bad things go. Sometimes it works to boost their ego, but if that sounds sarcastic, it is not worth it.

Boss Haters

Who they're: Boss haters often have personal issues which are hidden from those in authority. They refuse to be bound or bound by corporate staff. Boss haters resort to every means necessary until their patience is exhausted and they are eliminated. However, some of them are difficult to get rid due to union rules or skills.

How to deal? Perform a freeze-out. Try not to resist them. Avoid interacting with them. They can lose their energy if they are not around others.

Sliders

Who they are: Former Stars, The Sliders have always been Stars. They rely on their accomplishments while challenging their teams with apathy. They believe they have proven themselves worthy, so they remain in a protective bubble that nobody can burst. It is because they bring value and satisfaction to their company.

How to deal. Don't waste time complaining about Slider. You might be better off joining their fan club and showing respect for their contributions. Perhaps they'll become your mentor someday.

Pity Parties

They are the employees that have every excuse to not act. They are good at creating sympathy stories. Pity Parties understand how to let go of responsibility and give time to others.

How to deal: You should avoid these people and their pleas of help. As humanely and politely as possible decline their requests, regardless of what they promise.

Self-Promoters

They're always right and have a campaign for promotion. They make you feel bad and often steal your credit.

You must be patient and calm. You will get your much-deserved admiration. Do not let self-promotional people take the credit.

The best way to deal with difficult coworkers is to simply do your best and be a team player. Learn to adapt, cope and survive in a world that doesn't allow you to.

# Chapter 8: Is Depression Real?

"Oh, you just feel a little under-the weather." It will get better soon!

"Stop being such Drama Queen!"

"Grow up! Why aren't you being more responsible?

"You have so great things to be thankful for. So why aren't you happy about your life?"

"Come on. Why aren't you so upset?" This is not the end.

Many people have doubts about mental illness and trauma. They say it is a mild illness like small pox, which can cause serious problems in a person's life. However, they don't consider depression or that someone is suffering from an inner condition.

These are the kinds of comments that someone might say to someone who is feeling depressed. These comments can also be things that someone who is depressed might think, if they aren't aware of the severity and credibility of their problem.

These are two categories of people. The first topic I would love for me to discuss is "Is depression for real?"

It is very, very real. People who act depressed over the simplest of events or talk about how useless and empty they feel inside are not exaggerating. They really feel more miserable inside than they are letting on. They really feel as if their world is crumbling around and they are being depressed when they say they are feeling depressed.

Each person experiences ups and falls in life. There are moments when everything goes perfectly - like when our boss compliments we on a project, or when the baby smiles at us for the first and last time. These are the days where you will feel happy. You'll be happy, ecstatically happy, or tranquilly happy.

There are also 'bad days' that are quite normal. These days include those when you forget your umbrella and it begins to pour. Or when you arrive at your office only to find that your keys are missing from your home. These feelings aren't so bad that they have to be ignored. It's possible to get some sleep and a cup of coffee after a long, painful day.

But then there's the depression!

You're experiencing both the good days and the bad, trying to face every new challenge life throws at your. Sometimes depression appears suddenly and unexpectedly. You can feel like a disaster when you face the simple things in life. You feel like you want to go somewhere far away and die peacefully every time you encounter something negative in your daily life.

You've lost yet another pair of socks in the dryer.

You can't find your keys to your car, you feel completely lost, helpless and vulnerable.

Your newborn baby is crying and won't sleep. You hate this feeling and feel terrible for it!

Although your partner wants to be intimate with and for you, all you are feeling right now is tiredness.

It is not something you look forward to, but it is something that you fear.

You always feel sick inside and cannot stand others around.

You won't feel a constant sadness after you make a special family pie or miss your bus home. Sometimes, even a broken nail can make you feel so miserable that it lasts for weeks.

Depression is more real and common than other traumatic emotions. It is possible for depression to be present if such events are happening to you, or to someone close to,

For more information about depression and the best ways to cope with it, please continue reading.

# Chapter 9: Diagnosing Depression

It is simpler to explain depression by identifying its effects on one's life. Though the emotions are all different, they all fall under the same category: sadness. Living with depression can have a negative impact on your ability for society to function. It affects your ability to sleep, socialize and work, as well as your ability for normal daily living.

There are many factors that can lead to depression. There are many reasons why you might feel depressed, especially if you've had a major life transition. It could be the death or serious illness of someone you care about or loss of your job. These are just three possible causes of depression.

Don't waste another day or minute waiting for the feeling to be better. It doesn't happen automatically. You must actively seek out help and be open to change. Your happiness and wellbeing depend on how proactive you are in seeking help and guidance. Your positive attitude will help you overcome your problems and lead to a happier, more fulfilled life.

People with depression often find that it is difficult to do the same things as they did previously. It might be something you enjoyed doing but it suddenly becomes difficult to do. Some people feel lost, depressed, sad or even defeated. These are just some examples of emotions that people suffering from depression might feel. Depression can affect your mind, heart, soul and spirit. Your depression may look or feel very different from that of someone else. It isn't like a person. There are no red flags visible on the head. It can instead be identified by paying attention to the feelings and actions of someone struggling with depression or anxiousness, even though you may have to watch them.

Recognizing the Signs, and Implications of Depression

There are many signs that depression can be present in people you may know or have been diagnosed with. If you are not aware of their struggles, it is difficult for you to suggest they get help. Understanding depression is key to recognizing it and the effects it has on your life.

After you have recognized the signs, you can suggest or encourage counselling. The most obvious signs of depression are listed below.

Crying unexplainably or incoherently

An increase in or prolongation of periods of depression

Excessive anger or aggravation.

Cynicism

A lack of motivation or depleted energie

Resignation without cause

Guilt or lack of self worth:

It is difficult to stay focused or take decisions.

You are no longer interested what you once loved

Consistent pains or unexplainable aches

Stop repeating the same thoughts about ending your own life

It's possible to be depressed if you have or know someone who experiences the same symptoms. Once these signs have been noticed, it is important to act or seek professional help. Most people don't have the knowledge or resources to help them. Many resources are available to people who want to tackle this issue.

Take a look at the following:

For more information, contact your local mental hospital

Online search for counselors and private mental health professionals

Talk to people you know that have experienced or are coping successfully with depression

The following table can help you identify depression from just a bad mood. Although depression can seem like a normal part of life, many people who have it are suffering from chronic or persistent depression.

Bad Day Depression

Had a bad dream and couldn't get to sleep.

It is hard to find strength to replace your job when you lose your job over a decade ago.

You don't own anything to wear so you decide not to attend an event.

You're faced with too many challenges that can cause you to lose your appetite.

Are you tired of caffeine? You can't sleep. Many nights are sleepless.

Feeling guilty because your best friend missed their birthday.

Crying because you've lost your pet, suffered another type of loss. Crying when it is not necessary.

What happens after signs are detected? What is the next step? The stage of depression that you are experiencing will influence the answers. It might be easier for people to overcome depression early on. This is due to the fact that it may be the beginning of a negative situation or because the trauma is new. It is possible to recognize depression and take proactive steps to defeat it at the beginning.

There are steps you should take immediately if you or a friend is feeling or showing the symptoms of depression. Begin by taking care for yourself and encouraging others to do same. This doesn't necessarily mean you need to modify your medical plan or go for a more active lifestyle. Both may be important, but they aren't the only things to be done. The best thing you can do for yourself is to create a lifestyle of self preservation. This allows those with depression to maintain a healthy, happy, and long life. When you are at this stage, you will recognize the things that you most need to live happily and take action to make them happen. Engage in or participate with activities that distract or cause you to feel sad.

It is easier to overcome depression when you connect with your happy spot. This does not always have to be located in a particular place, but can also be inside. For happiness to be experienced, you only need something that makes your smile happy and makes you feel great about yourself. It can be overwhelming because you may not know how to get there.

The following activity chart will show you how to divide your day into different activities that are enjoyable.

Morning – The morning will determine the atmosphere for the rest of your day. Once you're awake, take the time to examine your true feelings. Reach out to them and learn why you have them. Enjoy a cup water, tea, or coffee while you meditate.

Listen to your favorite music. Decide to make the best of each day. Take the time to practice yoga or another relaxing and enjoyable activity. Get creative with your mornings by making it your own. Before you leave the house, stand in front of your mirror and think about three things you admire about the person looking at you. Next, think of two things you would change about that person staring back.

Mid-Morning -- Mid-morning can be a significant time for those who are suffering from depression. This is often when you start to focus on the things that are not working in your daily life. It is at this point that you often begin to compare yourself and others. STOP! Remember the positive things about yourself that you once admired before you left home. It's important to not be focused on what other people are doing. Instead, focus your attention on you and think of ways you could improve things about yourself. These are what really matter, but it is important to remember not to pressure yourself. There are only 24 hours in the day. If you don't achieve or make any changes today, tomorrow will.

Afternoons: Afternoons should only be used to recharge. Refuel and recharge your spirit. Take a stroll around your favorite neighborhood. Visit your favorite coffee shop or lunch spot. Spend the afternoon reading with children at their local library. These are activities that remind us of how vital we are in our lives.

Evening – The best time of the day to vent your emotions is evening. Negative events of the day must be ignored. Don't take anything personal. Most importantly, don't let bad situations or occurrences affect your ability to feel valuable. Be objective about what happened in the day. Then, move on to your evening. It might be helpful to tell yourself that whatever happens, you will deal. Now is the time to relax and enjoy your school or work day. Enjoy a night with friends, a movie with your partner, a concert or a movie night at the house. Relaxing baths with soothing music and long, relaxing soaks are great for ending the day. This will help you fall asleep faster and make your sleep more comfortable.

*Notice how morning and night are the largest times of day. These are the best hours to reset and reset your emotions. This will help you feel your best each day.

The Stages of Depression

Try to realize that not all medical professionals will recognize or assign stages for depression. It is important to remember that the common process for progression that a large number of people identify as stages. Before you feel any bodily changes, the way your thoughts and feelings change will be evident. It is not unusual to start blaming your self for things that aren't your fault or feeling down about life's challenges or problems. These common behaviors include eating more or less, staying up past midnight and pacing the floor.

As some people call it, the stages of depression can appear like this:

Observation – This is where depression can be diagnosed and the causes of it. You observe the changes you notice and can identify the symptoms.

Preparation - This stage is where you may talk to someone regarding your thoughts or feelings. You may begin to search for information or to consult self-help guides in order to understand what is happening in you life.

Take action and be proactive. Talk to a counselor, a doctor or other health care professional to get a professional diagnosis. You may be prescribed medication, or you might need to start therapeutic exercises. These measures can be used to promote relaxation and reduce stress.

How you Feel

Depression is a condition that causes mixed emotions. You may feel isolated from the rest of the world, lonely and demotivated. It is important to communicate or speak with others, establish happy and healthy relationships within your support systems, and surround yourself in people or things that make one feel happy and valued. These are all positive ways to overcome depression. It is important to remember that no one expects you be with or depend on anyone all the time. It is essential that you are able to enjoy activities on your own and not be sad or discouraged.

Take a look at these suggestions to make your alone time more enjoyable.

Be active

Depression can cause you not to be interested in your favorite activities and can even make you feel depressed. Be active at least thirty minutes a day. Go for a ride on a bicycle, throw a ball at your dog in the park, join a dance class, or do any other type of exercise you like. It is said that consistent exercise will improve your mental and physical mood. It can help with depression that many people feel. Exercises that involve active movement can help improve mood and lower depression symptoms.

Relax

Depression sufferers often feel stressed or worried about outside factors for a large portion of the day. It's time relax. Meditation is a great way to relax the mind and get your body in a relaxed state. It helps to break the cycle of negative thinking. There are many styles of meditation. You might consider enrolling in a class. Or, if it's easier, watch a video or meditate with a professional on television.

Adopt a Pet

Pets are as loyal and loving as the people they love. They are great at helping people overcome depression and loneliness. The responsibility of caring for a pet can make you feel empowered and in control. If you have suffered from depression, it is a good idea to start with a smaller animal. This will prevent you feeling guilty about not walking the dog, trimming the cat, and taking care of other responsibilities regularly. Your life will be filled with fulfillment if you have pets.

Volunteer

It's a great feeling to give your time to those who are most in need. Volunteer in your school, at work or community. Volunteering can bring you satisfaction and help organize an otherwise chaotic lifestyle. You will feel more self-confident and happy when you see others appreciate your efforts. You can volunteer for as little as two to five hours a month and you will start to notice the changes in your mood. It is important that you keep it light and not feel obligated.

Join a Book Club

Do you enjoy reading? Books are a great way of expressing your inner happiness. If you're a reader who prefers to read on your own, you can pick up an inspirational or motivational book. No matter whether you're reading for enjoyment or self-improvement. Engaging in a storyline which encourages positive emotions is critical.

Music is the best!

Do you love to dance and music? Perhaps you have a favorite song or artist that has been a while since you last listened. When you feel down, download a few of your favorites songs and listen whenever it suits you. Get out there and dance to some of your favourite songs. You are allowed to dance outside in the sun or in the rain. The idea is to turn up your music, move around and have fun.

How Depression Can Impact Your Body

Depression can change your physical appearance, just like it can your emotional state. You may notice signs in your body that you are suffering from depression, even before the symptoms get too severe. The result of trauma or temporary symptoms may cause these signs to persist for long periods. You may be experiencing severe depression if your sadness lasts longer than two to 3 weeks. Another condition that may be associated with symptoms of depression is Post-Traumatic Stress disorder (PTSD) and bipolar disorder.

Person who has five or more symptoms in two consecutive weeks is diagnosed with depression.

Mood of sadness or feeling defeated most days. Tiredness without cause

Unable enjoy favorite activities.

Extreme weight reduction Extreme weight gain

Feeling low self-worth.

It is time to put aside any thoughts that may be causing you to consider suicide.

Depression has an impact on not only your personal life, but also the lives around you. Depression can affect your relationships at home, at work, and within your social circle. How has depression changed your life? Maybe you haven't noticed that there are changes happening in your life.

Sufferers with depression may also experience these effects.

Depression could be the root cause of your uncontrollable feelings, emotions, and changes within your body. Before these symptoms become life-threatening and more severe, it is important that you seek professional help. How your body reacts emotionally can impact your body's performance. For happiness and health, it is worth taking the initiative to get regular physical and mental check-ups.

# Chapter 10: Creative Ways To Make You Happy

The people with the highest creative potential tend to be the ones most likely feel depressed at one point or another in their lives. There are a few factors that can explain this. If creative energy is not allowed to flow, it turns against us and causes us to see the worst. We must use our imaginations creatively in order to prevent them from turning against ourselves. Our imaginations need to flow, and be creative to keep them healthy.

For our thoughts and emotions, creative passions can be a great way to get out of our heads. A creative nature is both a blessing, and a curse. It is a fact that most people don't have a lot of creative freedom because employers, corporations, and business owners often push for more micromanagement. If you are lucky enough have a profession that allows you to be creative, then take advantage of this opportunity. If you find it difficult to be creative, or if your job doesn't inspire you, it may be worth pursuing your passion for creativity on your own.

Here are some great creative activities that can help you instantly transform your sadness into creative joy.

1. Do things you're good in.

A passion that you are good at is one of the best ways to instantly boost self-esteem. It will immediately make you happy, and you will feel great about your chosen field. If you are unsure about what you might be good at, you can look back at school or your childhood to see if there was a passion that you had.

2. Write.

Writing is therapeutic. You can write in journals or create blogs. You can write about your feelings, your pains, the joys you have, and even your dreams. You can also make your writing a profession if it is something you enjoy. Writing can be a great way to relax and express your creativity. It can also help you make some money. Or, you can write something that will inspire others. There is no limit on what you are able to create.

3. Paint.

Painting is a great way to relax and have fun, making it a good choice for people suffering from anxiety and depression. Painting can calm your mind and help you relax. It is therapeutic to paint. All creative endeavors help relieve tension in the unconscious mind and reconnect us with a source creativity that takes us out of our heads to bring us back into joy.

4. Try origami.

Origami is a paper-based art that allows you to make many different things. Like painting or writing, origami has therapeutic properties. It will instantly improve your self-esteem. You'll feel better about learning, design, and the entire process.

5. Every day, achieve one important task.

Depressed people will never feel the need to do anything. To motivate yourself, take one small step every day. It is possible to do one important thing each day. It can boost your self-esteem and give you a sense if you are successful. Make a "to-do list" every day. Keep it simple and manageable - no more than three items. Prioritize the most valuable task. This will allow you to feel dopamine increase, which will lead to a significant boost in your motivation and self esteem.

6. Do something for someone else.

Depressed people will find it hard to get up or rise early in the morning. It can help you feel instantly better. You can make a difference by getting up earlier and dedicating some of your time to helping others. Random acts or kindness can instantly make someone feel good. You can:

Ask your parents what's going on. This will instantly make their day.

Get coffee with your best friends and make it a payment. This is a great way for you to meet someone you like.

Help a homeless person by buying them a hot meal. This will instantly make you feel good, and it will also remind you that you are fortunate and that there are many things you should be grateful for.

Any random act or gesture of kindness

Again, these suggestions are just suggestions. Perhaps you prefer the feeling of piano keys under you fingers, a trowel at your side as you plan your garden, or the right combination and seasoning to turn you into a great cordon blue. It might be the grease and shine of repairing a Harley Davidson motorcycle engine or the harmony from your choir. There are many creative possibilities. You can bring your own unique flair to any situation. Spend some time imagining what you like! Then, start taking the smallest and easiest step that you find most enjoyable.

Doing good things and creating beauty will help you feel great about yourself. But it is essential to continue doing this on regular basis. This means that even if you feel better, you need to keep at it. As with the other easy, fun steps in this book: the more you do them the more joy you'll have and the greater your ability to cope with difficult situations.

Kindness and compassion instantly take you out of your head and into the heart. This allows you to connect to the world and other human beings. One of the most surprising things about sadness and depression, is that it allows you to better understand the deepest sufferings in life. That understanding can be used to help others. You don't have to be a martyr. Instead, take care for yourself and do not let others suffer. This will exhaust you quickly and you won't have the ability to help anyone.

Smile today and bring a smile onto someone's face. Make a child giggle, or make a baby smile. Help an old lady cross the road. Be kind and compassionate to others. This is a wonderful way to be more fulfilled and you will feel stronger, wiser and more loving.

# Chapter 11: Maintaining a happy attitude in life

The previous chapters covered the key strategies and techniques needed to be happy seven day a week. It would be a good idea to summarize the main points made in the book. Below are some of your questions as you go about your quest to find genuine happiness.

Is happiness something you choose or something that happens randomly? Many people mistakenly think that happiness is something that comes randomly. It does not. Happiness is something we should strive for. It is a decision you make and something that grows organically. You must be proactive about seeking it. Find your inner peace. Experience life outdoors. Follow your passions and work hard to achieve them. Be a good friend and partner with your family. Look for happiness, you'll find it.

Why is happiness harder than despair? This is all down to what each individual believes and holds dear. There are many possible ways to react in any given situation. Each response is a reflection of the values and beliefs we hold dear. The key is to design a system that will allow for discipline, self control, and the ability to see the positives in every situation.

Can happiness ever be quantified? There are many definitions of happiness. Therefore, it is difficult for anyone to give a universal measurement. Some people consider happiness to be tangible wealth. Others define happiness as an inner peace and calm. This is a mental and emotional state that is free of worries and stress. There are many variations, but happiness can be defined as a feeling of satisfaction with yourself and others.

Is happiness possible? You can achieve happiness if only you are determined. It is something you need to work for. You can be happy by removing all negative emotions. It's about strengthening your perspective on yourself and your relationships with other people. It is possible to achieve happiness through mutual experiences.

Can I be happy? Every person deserves to feel happy. It's your choice to be happy. However, it depends on your outlook and how you think.

It is possible to find happiness. All that is required to attain happiness is willpower, perseverance, and the belief that things will turn out in your favor.

# Chapter 12: Can I Stop My Own Depression

The answer is a clear, affirming yes. Some people may believe that mental health professionals are the only ones who can help with depression. These professionals can offer different treatments for depression.

I would strongly advise you to contact the nearest emergency department if you feel like you are going to commit suicide or endangering others. This is a true emergency.

If you feel depressed or anxious, I urge you to contact a mental-health professional.

However, anyone who is suffering from depression can still follow the guidelines in this book to get rid of it.

Unfortunately, many people don't find relief when they see mental health professionals. You should still try it. It is like shopping to find a counselor. It's like shopping. You must shop around until you find the right person. The best thing for you is to find a professional who can help you.

However, many people depend too heavily on antidepressants that can be easily found as a "fix-all" potion. But they can have unpleasant side-effects, and often don't work well. Anti-depressants are a common choice. It's understandable. They are looking for a way to resolve their problems, which is a good thing.

Sometimes people require antidepressants in order to feel better until they are able to resolve the root causes of their depression. The problem is that many people start to believe that depression is caused by something they don't know how to fix.

This book will guide you through the process of getting rid of depression as well as how to become healthy in mind and body.

What can you do to help yourself from depression?

You only have to be open to changing your behavior in order for depression self-help. You'll learn how. This is not difficult work. Change your life now.

Making New Habits

We all have our rituals and habits. These habits have led us to where are now. They define us, who we are and what they have made of us.

When I was depressed, my daily habits revealed that I had a set routine that made it easier to feel down.

I can say that my depression was caused by my lifestyle:

I ate poorly (by which I mean non-nutritiously).

I stayed awake until well after midnight, even though it was necessary to get up for work or care for my children on the weekend.

I let most of my body be inactive for the majority of the day.

I often contemplated the things I hadn't achieved enough of (successful, money and love, for example).

I thought about all the misfortunes in my life: loss of job, marriage breakup, loss to a child, etc.

I slouched on the floor, and then looked down.

I frowned and/orcried often (I would sometimes hide and cry in the bathroom at my home or at work).

There is more!

Do any of these sound familiar or not? It's worth taking a moment to reflect on the behaviors that are contributing to your depression.

There may have been some chemical imbalance in my brain. Even though I tried to take the most effective antidepressants on the marketplace (and I tried many), I was not able to alter my very effective and successful habits to avoid depression.

I can confirm that it wasn't a hormonal imbalance. I actually felt happy and fulfilled. There was no need for meds. It was a shift to new habits.

If I can do this, anyone can. You'll learn how.

How to Create Your Map

Make a list of habits that will lead you to your goal. I will show you how to create customized habits for you.

First, you have to map your self. You need to know where you are at the moment and where you want your future. Let's begin by recognising your current habits. Here's how. The following is what you should write on a sheet of white paper.

1. Write down what you feel. Write down the feelings you are experiencing. Be specific!

2. Next, take a look at your list of daily routines. These are the habits you follow

to feel those emotions. Be specific! You'll find many rituals to support your feelings. If you take the time to reflect on these rituals and write them down you will become more self-aware.

Take the time to be thorough from the moment that your alarm goes off until you fall asleep. Take the time to think about it. Be precise!

Take a look at all the habits you are practicing every day. Make a list. Write down all the activities you do every day. List what thoughts you have throughout each day.

Here are some questions you can answer. Answer these questions:

Your Mind

What do you want me to focus on? Do I focus on the good or the ugly in my life experience?

Do you dwell on a difficult situation? Is it just one? Write them down.

Is my self-talk negative or positive? What are my thoughts?

Your Physiology

What can I do about my physiology and depression?

Do you cry?

Do I slouch

Do you frown or look down

Am I grumpy

Your Personal Habits

Are you guilty of eating junk food, skipping meals, or eating too much?

Do you spend your entire day staring at the computer at a desk?

Do I sit idle or do I exercise? What is the best time to sit or do you exercise?

3. Write what you want. This is your dream destination. Would you want to live a normal day if there were unlimited resources? Make sure you are specific

Unlimited resources are the same as unlimited resources if money were not an object or your health, relationship, etc.

It is about how you feel and live your life. Real experiences, not materialistic needs. Be very specific!

Picture a Tuesday that your children and you both go to school on. What is the ideal way that you would spend a Tuesday? You don't need to do all the crazy things that would kill you every day. Do the same thing every day, but in a way you'd love to experience.

Your entire day: From getting up in the morning to getting back into bed and sleeping, to your final exit. How would it be to have a daily experience like this? Make sure to be very specific!

Here's an illustration:

"I want the ability to smile, feel refreshed, and that I feel like a new day is dawning brightly and beautiful upon me, full with possibility and enjoyment.

"I get up, get dressed and go for a walk or run on beautiful terrain. I feel the energy and strength of exercise strengthen my body and renew my mind.

"I want to have fun with my husband and laugh at the jokes and silly things my children do."

"I want to feel pride and energy at work. I also want to know that I've been successful in my craft."

"I'd like to meet up with good friends for lunch, have meaningful and entertaining conversations, and eat healthy food.

"I want the opportunity to pick up my children after school and have a pleasant time outside with them, laughing at all their silly games and preserving their innocence."

"I eat a nutritious, tasty, and healthy dinner with my loved ones, and we share the events of the day, and we also laugh at each other's stories."

"I get up in the morning and grab a book. I read for a while while sitting by my husband.

"I go down to bed in a serene and clean bedroom, feeling satisfied, tired, and certain that I have made my contribution to my loved ones, friends, society, and that I am grateful for the chance."

"I fall to sleep tired, but I feel happy and peaceful."

Be as specific as possible. If possible, include more. As much as you can, every moment of the day. The more detail, the better.

To create the best experiences, force yourself to stretch your imagination. This can go on as long as you'd like. The sky's the limit!

You're doing great! Keep going. Next, write the following.

4. What are some habits that I "should" adopt to have the experience I want?

These habits can be difficult, but I'm sure you'd love to have them. Be precise!

Define a life you would love to live. Include your facial expression and body posture frequently.

Be specific about which habits and rituals are necessary to live the life you want. Important is how your body and facial expressions are arranged. Remember that mind and body are linked.

These questions can help you answer these questions:

What do I do, and what do I think about when I wake? Do you smile and consider the blessings I have?

What should I do about my facial expressions, body posture, and body language throughout the day. Straighten your spine by sitting straight. Keep your eyes open for the beautiful sky. Look up often and notice the beauty of the sky.

Do I exercise? What kind of exercise are you looking for? What would you do to love exercising? Is there a childhood sport that I loved? How many years? How often and at what times do I exercise?

What should I do or think about at breakfast?

What do you discuss with your family?

What are my facial expressions and body posture?

What do they think of when I arrive at the office? How do they behave and how do I interact with others during my workday?

What do I do to eat lunch?

What are my facial expressions and body posture?

What do I do for fun and to think about when I'm done at work and go home?

What do I do when my house is empty?

What do you suggest I do for dinner, and tell my family?

What are my facial expressions and body posture?

What can you do to relax and go to bed at night?

This is a great chapter that will help you to identify positive behaviors.

5. Post Your Desired Habits. For 30 days, take your list of desired behaviors and place it somewhere that you can see daily, like your mirror or bathroom wall.

Copy it and place it at work

Start again after you have failed one day. Habits die quickly if they're not followed. You can keep going until the tasks on your list become second nature, and then they will replace your old habits.

Yes, your circumstances in life have not changed. It is possible that your marriage is still rocky, or that your loved one has died, but these are just two of many factors. You can make a list right now to see what you can do.

Your life will gravitate towards positive things. It is important to think positively in your life. Keep going back to your list and keep practicing it.

These are great ideas! Try them. It's fun to play around with. Add it and make a note of it.

For years you've been trying to get depressed. Let's pretend we don't know how to be depressed. What's the worst possible thing that can happen? You might still be depressed.

I guarantee that you will experience a life-changing transformation if you follow the advice on your list.

You'll start to see the changes happening slowly. One at a.m. Have you ever felt deja vu before? Did you ever think of someone you hadn't seen for a while and then suddenly meet them in an unexpected way.

This is called the power of attraction. This ability is common to all. We can attract what we believe we can with enough persistence. If you do it enough time, you will eventually become a pattern.

Only habits can be created if they are practiced for at least 30 days. Breaking a day is easy. Just reset your calendar and start over for the next 30 days.

This is called the law of attraction. It's real. It's something that is often discussed on television and in movies like "The Secret."

Now that we know the law, I want to share some tips and tricks that will bring happiness to your life.

# Chapter 13: Challenges of Negative Thoughts

Behind a smile

You may think that depression symptoms are the same as people who feel sad, hopeless. They also look depressed, lonely, apathetic, and helpless. This is not always the truth. Depression can sometimes go unrecognized because it is complex and concealable.

How can this be? This case is unusual in that the depressive symptoms can be atypical. These people are depressed daily, even though they seem happy and active. This type of depression is known by several names, including somatization, hidden depression, smile-making depression and masked depression. It is not covered in current psychiatric classification systems (DSM IV or ICD 10). However, many clinicians recognize the atypical form. It's a clinical phenomenon that can be found in any age. The most common time masked depression is experienced is after middle-age.

Living with smiley depression is the ability to accept that people who suffer from depressive thoughts may not lose their day-to-day functioning. They may continue to have a full-time job and participate in activities such as sports or social events. Their smiles are fake and frozen. This is a defensive mechanism used to hide real sadness and disappointment. Most people don't see this and insist "on being fine."

Even with their high achievements, brain sharpness, social life, and social life, gifted adolescents may struggle with depression symptoms like low self esteem or sleep disturbances. These teenagers feel different from others. Although they tend to say there is nothing wrong with being different, their subconscious beliefs about vulnerability and sharing feelings are a source of vulnerability. Their parents also notice a decrease in emotional responsiveness.

These hidden talents can be found in anyone regardless of age.

They need to hear that they are okay not being fine. Remember that it can be hard for friends and family to understand that someone they care about may have masked or hidden depression. Additionally, they can be furious at the mere mention of the "d" word. They may try to convince your that you are exaggerating. They know inside that you are correct.

Here are some ways you can help your friend/relative.

* Approach them with understanding and compassion

* Do not argue with them about how good they are.

* Speaking from your heart.

* Share your emotions.

* Describe any past experiences that made you vulnerable and helped you.

* Give them the option to choose a practitioner they are comfortable with.

Remember that there are ways to treat this type. A clinician who is familiarized with the clinical diagnosis won't underestimate the severity of a situation. He will recognize the subtle signs and symptoms, as well as the negative thinking that often characterizes depression.

What is negative Thinking?

Negative thoughts are an indicator of depression. It is characterized by feelings of helplessness (grace, guilt), worthlessness, low self-esteem, and feeling helpless. People suffering from depression are often faced with many difficulties. They have difficulty seeing their own perceptions and relationships. These cognitive distortions are thoughts developed from thoughts that were not triggered by events.

They are able to "pop up", and they can torture anyone suffering from this condition.

People can feel hopeless, helpless, and depressed when they are flooded with automatic negative thoughts. Although people try to be positive, it's hard. People who are depressed don't have to be negative. Positive thinking is not an automatic process. According to their perspective, the majority of negative thoughts seem to be realistic. These thoughts cannot simply disappear in a magical manner.

Concerning negative thoughts it is suggested that either avoiding or fighting against them is not always the best option. There are times when it is useful to challenge these annoying thoughts. It is better to end them than let them continue if you feel weak or insecure.

Cognitive Behavior Therapy, one the most powerful forms in psychotherapy, states that people suffering from depression need to work on their unhelpful thinking.

Cognitive Behavior Therapy claims that this is the case

Thoughts, beliefs, and perceptions can affect emotions. The emotions we feel when confronted by a situation can come to the surface. What we believe about the situation and how it is interpreted can have the greatest impact on our final reaction. If you make mistakes in your work you might feel disappointed and frustrated. The automatic

One negative thought that you could have been able to think of was, "Im useless."

Depression sufferers will find relief by understanding why their negative thoughts appear and how to spot them. People suffering from depression will feel better if they are able to cope with their negative thoughts. Cognitive behavior therapy is a way to overcome negative thoughts.

The best way to combat negative thinking is:

Be open to all negative thoughts.

It is possible to find the causes of your thoughts not being true to reality.

Reframing negative thoughts into realistic ones

Ask for help from people who are familiar.

Asking for expert CBT guidance from a clinician.

Beware of thinking traps

People who are depressed don't do it because they want to, but their brain and past life experiences can cause them to think negatively. First, recognize the signs of depression.

Here are the top five most common thinking traps.

* Overgeneralization:

"Mum is angry that I was late. She hates on me. She won't allow me to go again." People tend to make general conclusions about events without considering all evidence. They will focus on the negative aspect of a story, using words like "never"," "always", etc.

* The thinking of "All or Nothing"

"I made mistakes."

Although there are many shades of color, most people see the world in black and white. They believe that everything is right or wrong, and good or evil. They don't see that there may be a middle ground. The primary characteristic of this distortion is the insistence on the negative side. Focusing on only the negative aspects of an event and ignoring all the positive aspects can distort reality as is.

You might be unhappy about your work

Although it can be difficult to ignore the fact that it is a lucrative job, you cannot deny its positive impact on the environment.

* Exaggerating or expecting a disaster

"My boyfriend isn't texting me."

"He is about to leave me."

People fall into this trap when they overestimate the effects of their actions. People see the worst possible outcome and overestimate the consequences. They are afraid to wait for these scenarios and live with anxiety.

* Mindreading:

"I am ugly."

"I went along to a birthday party and when I got inside, I saw men thinking about how ugly my skin was." People believe that other people know what they think or feel about themselves. They believe they are able to read their minds by using their intuition and make quick decisions without having any proof. They are often unable to read the actions of other people. In their mind, speculations have become certainties.

* Fortune telling:

"There is no need to go out with Tom."

"He will refuse me."

In this example, people make predictions about the future, acting as fortune-tellers. They believe that their past behavior will influence their future judgments.

* Emotional Reasoning

"I feel hopeless."

"There is no answer to my problems."

Sometimes intense feelings are influenced by circumstances. These facts cannot be confused with feelings. They believe it is more logical for feelings to be based on thoughts. This cognitive distortion is where people base their thoughts on the feelings they feel.

* Personalization

"Luke seems sad."

"It must've been something I did to disappoint him."

People will blame others for something that wasn't their fault. This is not the reality. They become involved in any negative event. They believe everything around them is a repercussion of something that they did.

* Labeling

"I made a mistake."

"I'm a loser."

In this instance, people are able to identify their own shortcomings. They often label themselves or their behavior in a negative manner.

* "Should" statements

"I shouldn't put off the realization of the project."

"I am useless."

People use words such as "should"," "ought, or "must" to criticize themselves and others. This can lead to anger and guilt. People fall for this thinking trap because they are morally provoking others to act in a way that is unmoral. It can also lead to guilt or feelings of inadequacy.

Challenging Thinking Tricks

Cognitive Behavior Therapy looks at how people who are suffering from depression believe that their perceptions of a situation are biased by automatic negative thoughts. Challenging negative thoughts isn't about changing one's way of looking at things. It's about keeping a realistic view of life and setting realistic goals. Not all people will feel happy or disappointed when they challenge negative thoughts. It simply means that, despite the negative emotions, people can recognize differences between situations and feelings and try to resolve them. Let's now see an example of how CBT challenges negative thinking. Paul suffers with depression and claims that he is a failure at every task he undertakes. He feels sad, unworthy and hopeless. It is crucial to encourage him and remind him that he can do anything. The next step is to let him know that he can fail at things, but that he has great abilities.

Positive thoughts can be overcome by self talk. If you feel overwhelmed or compelled to think negative thoughts based on emotion, it's time to stop and ask yourself: Are there mind traps? Which one are you?

Is there evidence that the thought is real?

Is it possible for emotion to be confused with facts?

Am I sure?

What would I say if a friend had the same idea?

Is this my first experience with this?

Is there a better scenario than this?

What's your worst nightmare scenario?

Can I manage the worst case scenario?

Do you wonder if I am right or are you certain?

This is how you can control your thoughts and not get overwhelmed. It may seem difficult at first. Depending upon the severity of their symptoms some people think it's impossible or very difficult. They are relieved that they can continue to practice this daily and experience the first positive outcomes.

Cognitive Behavior therapy defines negative behaviour as challenging.

Recognize the negative automatic thought.

You can refute negative automatic thoughts by using real evidence.

Alternative positive explanations

To control your thoughts, use distractions

Contest the underlying beliefs.

Let's not forget a negative thought. Tony was devastated by a workplace mistake and his boss called Tony to discuss it. Tony believes he has no skills and cannot do anything.

Negative thought: "It is useless!" Tony sees himself as ineffective. He is sad, ashamed and disappointed.

You can disprove negative automatic thoughts using real evidence. Tony made mistakes at work. Actually, he committed the mistake because he was simultaneously working on several projects. To encourage him to not be occupied with too many projects simultaneously, the boss made mention of his mistake.

Alternative explanation: Although he is capable and capable of taking on projects, he can't manage to do multiple projects simultaneously. His boss remarks about Tony's job. This is because he believes it will allow him to do his best.

Be clear about the core belief: I am useful. I don't have enough spare time so I can't do too many projects. Humans all make mistakes.

Refusing to accept negative thoughts is not as easy as it sounds. You shouldn't be discouraged or feel worthless if you try it or someone else. Depression is a serious mental condition. A CBT expert can help you to tackle all of your negative thoughts. Participation could include training your family on positive thinking, or family therapy.

# Chapter 14: How Friends and Family Deal With Anxiety

It's difficult to deal avec family members and friends who suffer from depression or anxiety. You cannot just ignore it and move on in your life. It would be better if they put the problem in the background. However, that could result in them resorting to drugs and alcohol to fix the problem.

There are many methods to support your family members who are experiencing anxiety disorders or panic attacks.

These are some of the signs that could alert you to someone who is anxious:

Seems restless.

Avoid situations that may seem ridiculous

It is time to think about future catastrophes

Can't seem ever to throw anything away

117

Is reluctant leave the house

Spends too much time organizing things

Is it difficult to sleep or stay asleep?

Has trouble concentrating

Frequent nightmares

Avoid situations or places that could be reminiscent of a past trauma event

You are plagued with self-doubts

Severe episodes of shakiness and distress.

Keeps you alert for possible dangers

It's okay to criticize

Everything is very important to me

Superstitions seem to plague my life

Is too concerned about germs, contamination or dirt

It seems that she is unusually concerned with her health

Feeling nauseated, dizzy, or have aches/pains that are not explained?

Check that the doors are locked and the coffee pot is on.

Always worrying about everything

Has panic attacks

Seems scared of spiders.

If you're asked to go to social functions such as weddings or neighborhood functions, you might react with irritation.

You are familiar with them so you can tell if they are acting differently than normal. These are some signs. It's most likely you will spot it when they act differently than usual. If they have anxiety disorder, they will exhibit the same symptoms.

How to deal with depression in a loving one

Depression is easier than anxiety to manage.

It is essential that someone suffering from depression gets out of their house to take a walk and increase their serotonin level. The rainbow will appear if they continue to do this every single day for at least a week. They will experience a lift in their depression and begin to think rationally again.

It will be 10 times harder to get someone out of a depression condition. Here are the "Don'ts", when it comes to dealing with a family member with a depression disorder.

DON'T:

Don't let them discourage you.

Talk about depression with them if they do not want to.

Let it affect yourself (if you are not careful)

Expect quick turnarounds, especially when they have a medical disorder.

Don't feel guilty. They can make it better, if they really want to.

Do not give up! (Some cases can take more than a decade, and it might take a while)

DO:

It is okay to tell them they can speak openly with you without fear of judgment

Spend as much as you can time with them

Tolerating their transgressions is a good thing.

Get them outside. They will feel less depressed if they aren't thinking about their problems as much.

Be proud when you observe improvement.

Be yourself, and don't try being a psychologist.

Most people with anxiety and depression want someone to listen. If you don't know the best way to help them, just listening is enough. Encourage them to be active and don't allow them to fall prey to negativity.

Supporting a friend or loved one with anxiety and depression can help them return to their normal functioning lives.

They are both a challenge for those who suffer from one or the other of these diseases. They need every support from their friends and family. Try to solve their problems for them will only lead to more problems. Let them have your back until you can help them with their anxiety or depression.

If you don't have a degree, being there for them when needed is the best thing that you can do. If you're not able to solve their problems on your own, then it's best to refer them for medical attention.

There are many types of treatments that they can use to manage their anxiety and depression. Let's examine the types of anxiety therapy.

# Chapter 15: Postnatal Depression

This type is most common between pregnancy to two years after birth. Full-blown depressive symptoms may manifest in the form of anxiety, sadness, exhaustion or anxiety after pregnancy.

Depression can cause other physical conditions. This condition is often called co-occurring disorder. People with heart problems, such as those who have suffered from depression in the past, often experience severe cases. Recognizing such depression cases is critical and seeking immediate treatment is imperative. It can be a slowing factor in the recovery process of other conditions.

Now let us get a better understanding of depression and its symptoms.

How to Improve Your Self-Esteem and Fight Depression

Depression is very detrimental to your selfesteem. Thus, one of the best ways to fight depression is to boost your selfesteem. By improving your self-esteem you can manage depression better and even overcome it.

Here are some ways you can increase your self-esteem.

Let go of your inner critic. A self-critic can be a motivator to help you achieve your goals, to make others accept you or to bring you down. Find ways to eliminate the negative voices in your head. Replace them with positive self talk. Positive self-talk is uplifting and will help you feel more confident about yourself.

Keep short breaks. Too much can lead to depression. A short vacation can be enough to help you feel less overwhelmed. A short break can help you relax and unwind. The breaks are a chance to reflect on your achievements and determine what the next steps should be. It will be easier to overcome depression when you see that you have done a lot.

Never stop doing the right thing. You will see improvements in your self-esteem and results if you focus on it. But perfectionism can keep you from trying. Procrastinating will make you feel worse and you'll get less results. You can always improve.

Be positive when facing failures. You will stumble and fall every time you attempt something new. You don't have to stop there! Make yourself your best friend. How would your parent/best friend support you? Do the same thing for yourself. This will keep you from sinking into despair and allow you to become more constructive after the initial pains of failure start dissipating.

Be kind and compassionate to others. It is not only a way to treat others with kindness, but it also helps create a ripple effect that makes others think and act in the same way. Be kind:

Don't compare your self to others. You'll likely meet people who do better in certain areas than you, and even people who have more. Comparing yourself to other people is a destructive behavior that leads to failure. Be aware that you are better than others; this will help you to see your strengths and recognize what you have.

Other Treatment Options

There are many other ways to deal with depression. There are two other ways that depression can be managed:

Psychotherapy

Psychotherapy also known by the name talk therapy allows you the opportunity to identify and address the root causes of depression.

If you are able to find a good therapist, it will be possible to manage the depression and any other symptoms. You can also change your behavior patterns to help with this condition.

Psychotherapy is broad and can provide a wide variety of coping strategies. The most important thing is that you discuss all your concerns with your psychotherapist to create a plan which works for you. Psychotherapists will often use multiple techniques to help manage different types and types of depression.

What are the key points to keep in mind when you meet your first psychotherapist?

Here are some important points to remember when meeting with your psychotherapist.

Get started. Start by listing all the things that are bothering you and any issues you wish to solve. Take this list to your first appointment. It could include:

All symptoms of depression

Family problems

It is important to be open and honest with your therapist. Also, be sure to discuss your short-term or long-term goals. The therapist will tell you how long the treatment will last and when to expect changes. Do not be ashamed of sharing your concerns and feelings.

Make sure to check your list regularly and make sure you're making progress. Check in with your coach to confirm that you're reaching your goals. If you're not seeing progress, seek out a second opinion. It is important to take your time as results may not appear immediately.

Psychotherapy uses a variety approaches, including interpersonal, psychodynamic, and cognitive behavioral therapy.

Cognitive-Behavioral Therapy - CBT

This encompasses a range of strategies, techniques and treatments to conceptualize psychological problems such anxiety, posttraumatic stress disorder, addictions or stress.

CBT includes a combination or both cognitive therapy and behavioral treatment. Cognitive therapy examines how thoughts affect emotions. Behavior therapy focuses on changing your attitude towards challenging situations. CBT is a treatment that requires you to be involved in order to see tangible/best results.

CBT can be helpful in recognizing the thoughts and beliefs that trigger negative emotions. You will discover that certain beliefs and thoughts that can cause depression are false and ineffective, and how to change them.

An example is when you focus on a negative thought (like a mean individual) and apply the same negative trait everywhere (e.g. The human race. Another example would be to simply see things as good or bad. You might also be tempted to label yourself as worthless or useless. This could include beliefs such as, "If everything does not go as I expected, it'll be disastrous," or "Changing how I feel miserable is not possible"

CBT means:

Cognitive Restructuring

This technique recognizes how our thoughts, emotions and behavior all have an interdependent link. Any alteration to any one of these factors can affect the others. Anxiety or depression causes your emotions, thoughts and behavior to become more negative by feeding off each other.

Cognitive restructuring allows you change and recognize your thought patterns. This is an effective way to get rid of depression and anxiety.

How to use Cognitive Restructuring for Understanding and Changing Your Thought Patterns

Learn to identify and change the negative thoughts that affect your mood.

Calming yourself: This technique won't work if the thoughts or emotions you want to explore continue to upset you. Deep breathing can help you calm down. Simply take 10 deep breathes. Inhale deeply and expand your lower belly to allow your body to take in more oxygen. This will help to lower your heart rate, lower blood pressure, decrease stress, and slow your heart beat.

Analyze the situation. Identify the contributing factors.

A mood analysis is a way to note down the moods and moods you felt during the current situation. Do not try to express your feelings towards the situation. For example, a thought might be "She trashed mine work infront of my coworkers," while the mood could be insecurity, anger, and frustration.

Pinpointing automatic feelings: These thoughts are natural reactions you have when you are feeling the mood. Please also take them down. Consider the following example:

"My future in this company is at risk."

"But my work is excellent."

"No one is interested in me."

"Maybe that I am not good enough."

"She's so rude, arrogant."

Perhaps you will find that the most worrying thoughts are "nobody likes" and "maybe they don't think I'm good enough."

131

You should look for objective support evidence. Write down specific comments and events that led you towards the automatic thought. You could, for example.

"She detected a fault in one the scripts."

"Presentation did take place, but I was ignored."

Examine objectively contradicting information: Does it contradict your automatic thoughts or is it? Notify them.

"My customers like my work."

"When I trained in this particular area, it was my best class."

"The presentation was objectively sound. The work I did was original, well thought out, and real."

These statements are more rational than reactive thoughts.

Choose fairer and more balanced thoughts. Now you are able to view both sides of the issue, which will give you the information you need to make an informed decision. You could try different ways to ask the question, or if you are unsure, have a discussion with others. You can write specific thoughts if you come across a balanced opinion. In the above example, we can see:

"People were a little surprised or shocked at how she handled my situation."

"The manner she dealt with the situation was unprofessional."

"My work was okay, but not perfect."

"I am good at this work. My talents are highly respected and appreciated by many people."

Monitor your current mood. It's now possible to see the bigger picture and your mood should reflect that. Now, start writing down how you feel.

Think about what you can accomplish to resolve the situation. Sometimes you might find that by taking a balanced approach to the situation, you make it seem trivial and no need for you to take further action.

You can now make a list of positive affirmations and use them whenever you have similar automatic thoughts. Affirmations refer to positive phrases or statements intended to help you deal and overcome any self-destructive or negative thoughts. Let's learn more about positive affirmations.

Effective Affirmations For Depression Treatment

Affirmations are more effective when used in conjunction with other strategies, like visualization and goal setting. The following tips can help to create positive affirmations that help you deal with depression.

Assertations should be made in the present tense. This will help you believe the statement is true. You can use the affirmation "I am calm and happy" to get rid of sadness and depression. When you can focus on these words, you will gradually feel better.

Keep repeating: Repeat your affirmations at least once a day. Repetition of your affirmations gives them more power.

Include feelings in your affirmations: Saying or thinking affirmations with emotions makes them more powerful. Affirmations should be meaningful phrases. Get excited to see this change take place.

Examples of affirmations would be "I have the leadership position in my field," or "Im excellent at my job," or "I'm grateful for my team."

Medication

The treatment of severe or moderate depression with medication can be very effective. But, medications can have side effects that could not be applied to all people. Before you start taking any medication, make sure to talk with your doctor.

Medication includes the use antidepressants. Below are the different types of antidepressants.

Serotonin-modulators

Antidepressants - Atypical

Serotonin-norepinephrine reuptake inhibitors (SNRIs)

Selective Serotonin Reuptake Inhibitors (SSRIs),

Your doctor may suggest that you begin with lower doses and then gradually increase the dosage to limit side effects. If you have trouble falling asleep, your doctor may recommend antidepressants. Antidepressants may take time to kick in; you may notice a difference after a week.

The general recommendation is to continue taking antidepressants for at least six months, even after feeling better. This is in order to prevent the recurrence or recurrence.

Exercise

You can manage your depression symptoms by exercising. Exercises are a great way to find coping methods that you can use to help make feeling better a regular part of your life. Do at least 30 minute of exercise three times a weeks to see the effects on your serotonin.

Try weight training, martial arts or boxing to get in shape. Your attention will be shifted from your thoughts to the present moment when you are focusing on movements. That is what you want: to forget about all of your troubles and just focus on your present moment!

Do rhythmic activities that require you to move your legs and arms, such as walking, swimming, running and running. How does wind feel on your skin.

Keep your mind busy with an activity. It might not be very strenuous but it will help you get rid of depression.

Another way to manage anxiety and depression

These strategies will be complementary to almost everything we've discussed.

Maintain a healthy lifestyle: Eat balanced, healthy meals. You should include Omega-3-rich foods like flaxseed, walnuts, fatty seafood, and other Omega-3-rich foods in your diet. This is essential for your emotional health. Consume moderate amounts of starch, refined sugars, and starch. These foods can increase mood swings aswell as fluctuate in your energy level.

Get adequate sleep. Depriving yourself can lead to irritability or anger. Try to get up to 9 hours sleep every night. To do this, make sure your bedroom is as calm and peaceful as possible. This can be done by improving lighting, adding sweet scents of flowers and making your bed as comfortable as you can. You could also create a relaxing bedtime ritual. You can read, watch a show or listen to soothing tunes before bed. Avoid dramatizing scenes before bed, and limit your consumption of coffee or tea before bed.

Avoid alcohol and drugs. Substance misuse can lead to relationship problems, interfer with depression treatment, and make depression worse. Even if you're struggling with difficult emotions or traumatic memories, don't self-medicate by using drugs and alcohol. Particularly, panic attacks may be more common with alcohol and other drugs.

Remember to take your time and relax.

Exposure therapy. With exposure therapy, you are exposed to the symptoms of panic and in a safe and controlled setting. The goal is to help you learn better ways to manage them. To simulate panic attacks, you may be asked to emulate the feelings you have. You might be asked to imitate the symptoms of panic attacks such as moving your head around, hyperventilation, and holding your breath. Doing this in a controlled atmosphere will help you break the habit loop you have when panic attacks occur. You will have more control over your panic. It's simple to break the cycle of fear, especially with desensitization. When you are exposed to thoughts that trigger panic attacks (in a controlled environment), it becomes less frightening. Exposure therapy allows you to anchor panic-triggering thoughts with a word. You can then stop the panic attack before it escalates by using the word.

Exposure therapy is beneficial for anyone suffering from panic attacks, PTSD, or other mental disorders. You should seek professional guidance to avoid psychological breaks.

Not only can you use the information from this book to fight your depression, but you also have the option to help a loved one or friend with their battle. The following chapter will offer all the information necessary to help you do this.

# Chapter 16: Depression Cycle Assessment Test

Suicide and depression is not an option. Use the depression test to assess your current state. You will get a true assessment of your personal wellbeing.

An easy method to assess depression.

SABA Resources would analyze the assessment, and send you 25 interpretations of the statement of the report.

Modalities

I.Think carefully through the graph above and the questions that iiScore myself in sincere observation regarding self

iii. Multiplying column number and tick count

iv. Each answer should be listed in the box below.

v. Add all numbers from the category boxes to determine your percentage score

vi. vi.

vii. S n a p p o s t t h e e n t i r e a s s e s s m e n t to james 1 kom@ yahoo. To get 25 statements of the truth about your schedule, use Whats App 08035999220. Apply the results and get full expression in your personal definition.

SCHOOL OF ARTICULATION AND BEHAVIORAL-ALIGNMENT R RESOURCES (SABA RESERCES)

DEPRESSION CALCULATION TEST 101 (DCAT101). 08035999220

Date...................................

Names

NOTE: Don't be too objective with your rating of these 10 Performance Variables. You can score yourself at 100% and as low 10%.

Point Rigi D Loo k Unstab le Yield Floating Swimming Swimmin'g Absolute

Score 1 2, 3, 4, 5 6, 7 8, 9 10,

POINT QUESTIONS

in... 1 2 3 4 5 6 7 8 9 10

1. Overdo-As a thought, feel or FD imagine negatives.

2.. Do you find yourself too ensnared in dangerous thoughts and cannot stop thinking?

3.. Show your true values/ virtues by displaying them in other things.

4.. Overrun - Knowing what your mind is doing to you can help you gain inner control.

5.. Avoiding Overwhelm - How can you tell when you're overwhelmed by thoughts and ideas?

6.. Overpower-Decisionsubdued and leaving you helpless over a cause; calling for concern?

7. An overdose is a lifestyle today. Some aspects of the vices and deviations are now dominant.

8. Overreacting: Notice how you react to sudden negative withdrawals and incorrect acceptances?

9. Overview-You feel, think, and see worthless.

10. Overthrow-When everything seems hopeless and all activity is stopped.

CATERGORY SCORE

TOTAL SCORE PERCENTAGE

SCORE

S Distinction Extension Manifestation Comprehensi

on Attention Detention

OUTCO MES

0 - 30%

Superlative31 - 40%

Receptive 41 up to 50%

Indicative 51 = 60%

Assertive 61 - 70%

Aggressive 71-100%

Provocati

ve

The question on the 10 Cycles of Depression from Overdo to Overthrow is being asked. Each cycle comes with a 10 column. This allows for objective reflection and critical thinking. Each column corresponds to the same point score. So, the point score for 1-10 is the same as the column that precedes the 10 questions. Start each question. Before you answer each question, think about how well you are able to respond in ..." questions 1-1 0.

In accordance with their different meanings and critical messages, you can tick the question in front of you by marking it with a tick. End all the ticks with v. Make sure you address every question. Your total number should be 10 for each column.

How do you calculate the depression cycle's score?

i. Count the number and frequency of ticks appearing in each column

ii. Multiply the column's number by the number.

iii. Write down each answer in the appropriate column. A category score will show you how often you experience depression in a given mode.

How can I determine my percentage score

i. Add all of the figures from the category score box to get the total.

ii. Enter the sum of your total score as a percentage.

iii. Find the cluster where you belong, regardless of how high you scored. Recognize the cluster you are in.

iv. To find the relative gap analysis for depression, subtract your percentage score at 100%.

One thing to keep in mind

It doesn't matter which cluster you fall into, once you score a mark in column 3 (dull points score), you will be considered to have sensed the question. Count the questions in which you scored at least 3 points to see where you are likely to fall into depression. These conditions all need to be treated by professionals as soon as possible. These factors can explain why depression might be happening inside without people being able to see it. Quickly take your assessment and receive an immediate interpretation. You can also request intervention via prudence or proxy.

Reality checks about depression. Underlining assumptions Depression at all rates is a behavioral viral that must never and ever be enjoyed.

Within two weeks of its appearance, the depression track at 30 symptom was still within the sustainable range. Beyond 30% operation, there is a tendency towards a gradual downward slope of the depression track for the eventual catch. If you are experiencing depression beyond 3o%, it is time to start on the path of departure. A person with 30% of the experience may be able stand firm against depression. The reality begins to dawn and the emotional shock absorber' within every human being stabilizes the trend over the course of time to avoid a dip into the path of depression.

Dependent on the severity of symptom depression, a range between 31-100% could be considered unacceptable. This is your chance to conquer and manage depression.

# Chapter 17: Throwing Out the Old You

Sometimes you have to make an inventory of yourself if you want to build a better life. You have the best place to begin is with your possessions. I started with what was in my closet. I found clothes I hadn't worn in years. They were there because a partner wasn't interested, but they were always my favorite. I chose which clothes to keep, and which to discard. It's funny what happens to clothes. When you throw out clothing, it's like shedding old skin. It can make you feel fresh.

A good way to get therapy is to put all your old gladrags together in a plastic sack. If you don't like the stuff that you have been wearing over the past year, consider giving it away. It will give you two positive feelings. One because you are changing yourself and moving on. Two because you are helping someone special.

149

You can either donate your clothes to a local homeless shelter, or put your most treasured items in a store where they will sell them on a commission basis. Both of these options were possible for me. I made money from the best items while making others happy. I still remember feeling proud about what I had done when I left the shelter.

Clearing your mind is also something that you can do. You can get stuck in a funk sometimes because you live a messy life. Your mind is a mess. Your life is a disaster. By doing this you can clear away the clutter from your life and take a step towards overcoming depression. It's a good idea to do this in every room. You might also want to look at your hair and consider changing it. You can have your hair styled if you can afford it. Also, make sure you trust the staff at the salon to create the "new" look.

Other areas in your house that you need to get rid of include the kitchen. This is where you may have excess food or the larder. There may also be things you don't want to eat. Perhaps you lived in this house with someone else and it's time for you get rid of everything. Don't get bitter about giving away items you don't own. If you are able to accept visitors, simply move the items into cardboard boxes. To get around these, you can place the box outside and notify the person that they have a 24-hour window to collect it. If they do not show up, that's their problem.

Make a list of all your songs and get rid off the ones that make it difficult. You're trying to find joy, and it is not possible to do this if you keep adding more sadness to your life. These things should be put away. Keep an inspiring collection of music around that won't lead you backwards. Forward is the only way to go at this moment. I recall one song I used to listen to that could bring my to tears almost immediately. "Sorry, doesn't always mean it right" was it. I knew the lyrics and had it in my heart from the beginning. Like me, you must say "goodbye!" to all things that lead you deeper into depression. If you love the music, put it away. However, don't let it be a distraction from your efforts to get stronger.

It is common to believe that crying can improve your mood, but there are limits. You don't have to cry as much as you would like, and I did. You can have a good, long cry if something is making your unhappy. Then just let it be. Anything more than that is selfish. Believe me, I played that song and got every emotion out of it. It didn't make you a better person. I was capable of getting on with life and making better choices. I had had enough. I didn't need to feel like that anymore.

Friends who are often in tears get tired after a while. It can become very debilitating to have friends who insist on being in a depressive funk. It doesn't work and it is time to heal yourself. If it isn't then it's high time you got the upper hand and decided to figure out who you want. You are taking the step to freedom when you decide to move forward. This will allow you to discover new possibilities in your life that you didn't know existed.

One example is that although I never expected to be helping others with my own experience, I have. Even if the help you seek is not within this book's pages, maybe someone else is. Maybe they are ready to face depression head-on and embrace the new life. If this is you, do not give up.

It is important to read the book again and again until it is understood.

# Chapter 18: Postpartum Anxiety

New moms are often affected by postpartum anxiety. There is a distinct difference between postpartum sadness and also postpartum worry. Due to the rapid hormonal change that occurs in their bodies after giving birth, many women experience mood swings for approximately 4 days.

Postpartum anxiety was often ignored or disregarded by medical facilities for too long. This has actually changed over the years.

Postpartum anxieties can be severe and may significantly limit a mommy's ability care for her child. Postpartum anxiousness is the result of a physical alteration in the body's chemistry. Ecological tension such as inadequate rest, inadequate help for the child, as well other triggers, could increase the symptoms and make it difficult for the mommy.

It may take months to establish postpartum anxiety, although doctors believe it can be caused by hormone changes after giving birth.

Postpartum anxiety is a common condition that medical professionals tell new mothers. If they experience signs and/or symptoms, they should seek treatment.

- Sleeplessness and rest problems

- Singing effortlessly, or weeping at any time

Extreme sensations of shame

Extreme Sadness Sensations

If a woman is dating a man, and also he does nothing on the telephone, she presumes he is on a date with another woman. While this may seem unreasonable and unreasonable, the female still assumes it. Similar troubles are experienced by males.

Zoom.

Magnifying refers to making something seem more important than it really is.

Cognitive Treatment can resolve altered belief.

The parents of their children were anxious and had a tendency to make them feel uneasy about the world. According to cognitive treatment concepts, their anxiety is the result of a lack in confidence and also beliefs that aren't always true. They can get rid of their anxiety by changing their thinking and teaching them how to believe.

Cognitive treatment may also be a concern because dispirited people can have a different way of looking at the world, the environment, and even themselves. These altered ways of assuming are:

Electroconvulsive Therapy, also known as ECT, can be used in certain cases to treat severe anxiety and other forms of psychotic anxiety.

Some mothers are troubled by the thoughts and needs of their children.

Postpartum Psychosis refers to the idea that a woman may harm herself or her child.

If someone compliments you, then you can quickly focus on one defect and reduce that praise. You will be able to focus on one thing in the mirror and not the whole photo.

Postpartum Psychosis is similar in its nature to postpartum Anxiety, however it typically presents with signs or symptoms that are related to psychosis such as aberrations or ideas regarding harming a child, unusually illogical ideas, chaotic reasoning, or sensation got rid off or separated.

There are only 2 types of typical treatments for anxiety. They are mental therapy to address the psychological components of anxiety, and medicine treatment to treat the physical causes. While many anti-depressants are recommended by doctors, some may cause severe side effects. Some antidepressants are known to cause anxiety and self-destructive thought.

A mom and dad concludes that the teenager can't possibly have believed of this on her own. They suggest that she get the help of her buddies. The moms & dad conclude that the lady must make new friends as she has bad effects on all of her closest friends.

Approximate Reasoning.

If someone is intoxicated with approximate reasoning, they tend to reach a negative conclusion about a scenario that increases their anxiety or denies any other possibility.

There are many alternative and non-traditional methods to deal with anxiety. They are becoming much more popular. Alternative treatments might also be extremely effective in managing certain kinds of anxiety, such a Seasonal Anxiety or Postpartum anxiousness. Acupuncture, Homeopathy, and light treatment are all effective ways to reduce anxiety.

Continuous therapy helps individuals with anxiety to deal with their symptoms as well as find out what is causing their anxiety. Even though there is the possibility of relapses or even remissions in anxiety episodes, those who have been identified with it will still be at risk for having another episode.

Reduction.

A reduction does not mean that you should disregard your personal characteristics or care about your well-being. One is reducing their worth or self-worth.

Cognitive therapy, which is a type mental therapy, was created to help with anxiety. Aaron Beck, who was a psychoanalyst in the early 1960's developed cognitive treatment. Cognitive treatment is based around the concept that individuals with anxiety have a negative outlook on the world.

It doesn't matter what therapy is used to alleviate anxiety. The therapy should be recurring. Anxiety does not usually indicate a serious health issue. It's something that everyone has. If you have anxiety episodes, it is more probable that you will have additional.

Psychotic anxiety can be the most severe form. One in four people suffering from anxiety are diagnosed by the health center every year.

If a man assumes that women will not want him to date them because he doesn't have the ideal vehicle, then he will make sure to convince himself that he won't get any kind of day even if he has lots of other advantages that make him attractive to ladies. A lady may also think that she is not attractive to men due to her large nose.

- Fear.

A ticket for website traffic is issued to anyone who may be able overexaggerate. Instead, this individual will regard it as a severe life problem. It is a serious offense for a waitress to forget to serve a person's cold tea during lunch.

The best medication for anxiety treatment isn't always the most effective. However, some people find that a mixture of mental treatment and appropriate medications can really help with their anxiety.

- Anxiousness.

Discerning Abstraction.

Careful abstraction means that an individual focuses on one issue and makes a presumption.

Overgeneralization.

Overgeneralization can be when an individual draws a wide verdict based only on one event as well.

THERAPIES - ANXIETY THERAPIES

COGNITIVE TRAITMENT.

The best therapy for anxiety is mental therapy. It helps the person to develop coping skills and manage the triggers that lead to anxiety. People who suffer from depression can develop greater problem management skills that will help them to stop allowing anxiety to control their lives.

Psychotic Anxiety is the feeling of feeling unwell and also helpless. There are really only two kinds of treatment for anxiety that can be used in conventional clinical settings: mental therapy to help with the psychological elements of anxiety and medication to treat the physical reasons. Certain types of anxiety, such a Seasonal Anxiety or Postpartum Anxiety, may be treated with different methods.

Cognitive Treatment Objectives

Cognitive therapy is meant to address the psychological issues that are causing anxiety. It also teaches the individual how to see and analyze the world in a more precise way. The individual will definitely be less likely that they get involved in harmful thoughts that could lead to anxiety once they have actually corrected their reasoning.

Cognitive treatment can be extremely effective in treating anxiety psychologically. While cognitive treatment cannot directly treat the physical symptoms of anxiety it can reduce the impact of the psychological factors. People with anxiety who like to try different treatments often find that using cognitive therapy in conjunction with the other therapies can be a wonderful way to manage their anxiety.

Cognitive treatment can't be a quick fix. It is not uncommon for cognitive treatment to be long-lasting. However, cognitive treatment is an effective anxiety management strategy that has been proven to help with depression and other anxiety disorders.

Cognitive treatment may also aid individuals in improving their problem management skills so that they can manage the losses and anxieties that are part of everyday life. People who are able to deal with problems effectively will not be easily triggered by work losses, the death, transfer, or any other difficulty that could trigger anxiety.

Any type of anxiety treatment aims at reducing anxiety over time. Cognitive therapy is a crucial part of managing anxiety. Because it teaches individuals who struggle with anxiety how to alter their views and perceptions of themselves, it can be a vital part of any treatment. The signs of anxiety usually disappear or decrease when people see themselves in a healthier way.

LIGHT TREATMENT

Light therapy is more than just for seasonal anxiety. Light therapy is a proven treatment for many conditions like jaundice, psoriasis as well as jet lag. Light therapy can also be used to treat rest disorders, which could indirectly help anxiety.

Light therapy was first developed as a therapy to combat seasonal anxiety. Because organic light triggers serotonin production, seasonal anxiety can be caused by lack of sunlight. The use of light sources that are similar to natural sunlight will help bring the serotonin level back into balance.

Physicians can use light therapy to aid people suffering from persistent sleep disturbances or rest issues. They could help them reset their organic clock and get back into a natural sleeping pattern. The absence of sleep or sleeping disorders may be a reason for anxiety. Light treatment could also be used to treat anxiety.

Light therapy combined with other therapies like homeopathy can be an efficient and natural way to deal with seasonal anxiety. It is not effective for all types of anxiety but it can be helpful to those who suffer from periods.

A few people get sunburn after light treatment sessions due to the possibility of skin being damaged by the light. Light treatment could be too intense for some people, resulting in insomnia or sleep deprivation.

Light treatment can cause some anxiety, but it is possible to avoid them. Although light treatment can still be considered an alternative therapy for anxiety, it's one of the most common.

Non-seasonal anxiousness can also be managed with light treatment. While the process is still new, doctors often aren't sure just how effective light treatment will be in dealing avec non seasonal anxiety. However early examinations and tests indicate that light treatment might be as effective at dealing with seasonal anxiety as it was for seasonal anxiety.

PSYCHIATRIC THERAPY

Although psychiatric Therapy is not intended to be a recurring treatment for anxiety, it may be used when severe symptoms present or when cognitive treatment is necessary. An individual may choose to see a psychiatric therapist if they have ever experienced anxiety episodes.

Psychiatric therapies is another option for anxiety. These are often used together with cognitive treatment. Cognitive therapy addresses the person's ability to see the globe and place themselves on it. This will help them overcome anxiety in the long-term. But, at the same moment, the person needs assistance in dealing with the feelings of loneliness, despair, distress, anger, and even despair that can result from anxiety.

One of the downsides to Psychiatric Treatment is that sometimes the individual will really feel better because they are receiving lots of treatment as well the assistance from the specialist. The individual could even choose to stop the therapy. While Psychiatric Therapy treats the immediate symptoms of anxiety, an individual with anxiety needs to be able to develop the most effective problem management skills and attitude to manage life.

More than 80 percent of anxiety sufferers who go to Psychiatric counseling report feeling much better. If you want to combat anxiety for a longer time you will need Cognitive Treatment. This is to help with your unfavorable thoughts that may contribute to your anxiety.

For those suffering from severe anxiety, psychiatric therapy can be a lifeline. It gives them an outlet and a way to express the feelings of unhappiness and discomfort. Anxiety tends to feed on negative emotions, so it is difficult for an individual to get rid of the negative feelings and feel happier. The combination of psychotherapy and cognitive treatment with other therapies is far more effective for anxiety treatment than the use of only cognitive therapy.

# Chapter 19: Stress- and Depression- Relieving Diet Plans

We'll be looking at different foods you could eat to reduce your stress levels and depression. We'll also be discussing the habits and foods that you should quit if stress and anxiety are a problem.

What to eat

To be mentally strong and happy, it is essential that you eat nutritious foods. Here is a list to help you decide which foods you want.

Avocados

Avocados rank high in the list of natural foods that have the highest success rate at reducing anxiety and stress. Avocados are rich sources of B vitamins that can reduce stress levels and help with depression. They are also rich in monosaturated fats as well potassium which are beneficial for your body. A half-an-avocado per day with breakfast can help relieve stress and anxiety. It's a great idea to cut up bananas and mix it with avocado in the blender. Once it is smooth, you can spread it on bread.

Asparagus

Studies show that low levels of folic Acid in the brain can lead people to suffer from depression. This could actually be the main cause of depression. Asparagus is rich with folic Acid, which aids in naturally beating depression and stress. You can either cut it into smaller pieces or boil it in water. Then, season it with salt & pepper. As a side, you can saute them in butter and season with salt & pepper. It is also great for snacking.

Oranges

If you need to find relief from anxiety and/or stress, oranges will be your best friend. They are high levels of vitamin C, which can help reduce oxidative damages to the brain. Each morning, you can drink a glass orange juice. Make sure you don't add any sugar to the orange juice and just enjoy it as it is. You can even add it to a salad. Orange juice is a great way to boost your immunity and feel energetic.

Sweet potatoes

Sweet potatoes are delicious and very good for your mind. They are rich in beta carotene and other important vitamins, which is essential for your brain. You can easily cut sweet potatoes into small pieces to add to your salad. You can also add sweet potatoes to smoothies to increase the sweetness. They are also known as helping to reduce cortisol, which is a great way to reduce stress.

Almonds

Vitamin B2 is high in vitamin E, and vitamin E is important for immunity. You will feel more mentally stimulated and your brain will be able to work faster. To make almonds, soak them in warm water overnight. Peel them and serve them with breakfast. They can also be roasted and eaten as a snack. Almonds can be used in salads as a garnish by being cut into slivers. They taste even better when added to smoothies.

Salmon

Stress can be described as an increase or decrease in cortisol levels. You need to stop this chemical from increasing as much and consuming foods that can help you do it. Salmon is one example of such a wonderful food. Salmon is high-in omega 3 fatty oils, which help to reduce cortisol. Salmon consumption will improve your mental strength and fitness. Salmon is simple to prepare. Simply bake it for fifteen minutes and then drizzle with olive or season with salt.

Milk

Vitamin B is crucial for your mental health. Vitamin B2 as well as B12 are abundant in milk. This will allow you to be mentally healthy and active for long periods of time. Drinking milk twice a day is advisable. Once in the morning and before you go to bed at night. It is also rich with anti-oxidants which will nourish your mind as well as your body. It is also rich with calcium and proteins that will assist you in maintaining a strong physique.

Spinach

Spinach is a leafy-green vegetable that must be consumed if you want to get rid of stress and depression. Research shows that increasing magnesium levels can help lower cortisol levels. Just adding a few spinach leaves to your salads and curries can help increase the magnesium content. For a green smoothie you can add some leaves. Spinach is also high in vitamin B, which will help to lower the risk of oxidative injury to your brain.

Blueberries

Blueberries are high-in vitamin C, anti-oxidants, and vitamin A. The antioxidants in blueberries can help repair and protect brain cells from oxidative injury. Add them to your fruit bowl and enjoy them on a daily base. If blueberries are out of season, you can freeze them and use them whenever you need.

Oatmeal

Oatmeal is a good ingredient to add to your daily meals. It has chemicals that stimulate the release and maintenance of the happiness hormone. You'll feel happy and full of energy when you eat oatmeal. At least five oatmeal breakfasts per week are recommended. For a more power-packed breakfast, add milk or blueberries. For brain enrichment, you can toast some oatmeal to sprinkle over your salads.

What can you eat instead?

If you want to reduce stress levels and depression, you need to avoid certain foods.

Junk food

Junk foods are the first food you must avoid. These foods can have a lot of unneeded preservatives that can lead to stress. It is best that you stop visiting this place, even if it has been your home since childhood. Make healthy versions at home of these foods to reduce stress and depression. Make a meal planning ahead so you can quickly prepare the meal and don't need to order take-out.

Processed foods

Preservatives in processed foods are as harmful as junk food. Preservatives can be found in processed foods, which could cause you stress and depression. There are many processed foods, including chips, cookies, nachos or sauces. All of these items can lead to stress and anxiety. You can cut out all of these if they are not manageable. If possible, reduce them to a minimum. These can all be made at home.

Alcohol

To reduce stress and depression, you must avoid alcohol. These will only increase stress and depression. Drink as little as possible. Drinking alcohol at dinner should be limited to one glass. Avoid parties with your friends where you drink a lot. You will soon notice the difference, and you will feel more confident about yourself.

Smoking

If you are looking to overcome your stress and depression, you will need to quit smoking. If you have been smoking for a long period of time, you should quit. If you're having trouble quitting, you can visit a rehab centre. Stop smoking with people you don't know.

Drugs

The same is true when you use drugs. You should avoid drugs. You have to give up on these unhealthy habits and work hard to live a healthy, happy life.

Apart from this, it is important to be on-time with your meals and to get your bed at the right time.

These are the best recipes to get rid of stress

This chapter will focus on some delicious meals that will improve your mood and decrease stress.

Easy chicken soup

Ingredients

1 red onion, chopped

2 small carrots, chopped

1 leek.

14 of a leaf lettuce, chopped

2 chicken breasts skinned.

2 garlic pods, minced

1/2 tablespoon olive oils

1/4 teaspoon turmeric paste

1/4 teaspoon coriander paste

1/4 teaspoon cumin flour

1/4 teaspoon ginger Powder

Salt to taste

Salt to taste

Parsley can be used as garnish

Directions

Heat the oil in a small saucepan.

Add the chopped onions and let them turn translucent.

Add the chopped carrots, leeks, as well as the lettuce leaves to make it soft.

Make a paste by combining the ginger and turmeric with some water.

Add it to the carrot mixture, and mix well.

Now add the chicken breasts.

Allow the chicken to cook for about 10-15 minutes, or until it is soft.

Don't overcook.

Mix in the salt/pepper and simmer for 5 min.

Serve the soup into a bowl. Garnish with parsley leaves.

Cleansing tea

Ingredients

1 teaspoon lavender flower

2 tablespoons rose bud petals

1 bag of green Tea

1 cup of water

1 tablespoon honey

Directions

First, add the water in a saucepan. Then let it come to boil.

In a large cup, combine the lavender flowers, the rose petals with the honey.

Turn off the heat. Place the green-tea bag into the saucepan.

Allow it to steep for 5 min, and then pour it over the mix of lavender and rose petals.

Mix all ingredients well. Serve hot.

Salad made with tart fruits

Ingredients

4 tablespoons of coconut milk

1 tablespoon honey

1 teaspoon freshly squeezed lemon juice

1 tablespoon honey

1 teaspoon salt

1 clementine, chopped

1 pineapple chopped

1 banana, chopped

1 mango, chopped

1 green Apple, chopped

14 watermelon, chopped

2 tablespoons chopped fresh mint leaves

Directions

In a large bowl, combine the coconut milk and lemon juice with the honey and salt.

Add the fruits to a bowl. Next, drizzle the honey over the fruit.

Sprinkle the mint leaves on top, and then let the salad cool in the refrigerator for about two hours.

Simple brownie

Ingredients

1 cup unsalted, butter

1 cup dark chocolate, melted

3/4 cup plain bread flour

2 tablespoons coco powder

1/2 cup white Chocolate, Melted

3 large eggs

3/4 cup caster sucre

Direction

Start by heating the oven up to 375° Fahrenheit.

Mix together the butter chocolate, sugar, eggs and eggs.

Now add the flour mixture and coco powder. Mix until well combined.

Transfer the batter to a greased tray.

Bake it for 30-40 mins or until a skewer poked into the middle comes out clean.

Let it cool, then chop and serve.

Sweet potato and avocado salad

Ingredients

1 large sweet potato

1 large avocado

1 teaspoon lime juice

1/2 chopped red chili

1 teaspoon cumin flour

1 teaspoon honey

1 tablespoon parsley leaves

Directions

Begin by adding the lime juice with cumin powder, chili powder, honey and tossing it in a small bowl.

To soften the sweet potato, cut it into small pieces.

Take the avocado and cut it in half.

Use a spoon for scooping the avocado in its interior and placing it in a container.

You can cut the scoops to make squares.

Add the pieces of sweet potato to the bowl. The honey chili dressing can be drizzled over the bowl. Toss together.

Salt can be added as needed.

It can be garnished with the parsley, and then eaten fresh.

Easy salmon bake

Ingredients

3 pods garlic, minced

5 tablespoons olive oleic oil

1 teaspoon basil leaves

Salt to taste

1 teaspoon lime juice

1 tablespoon fresh chopped parsley

2 fillets salmon

Directions

Start by heating the oven up to 375° Fahrenheit.

Add oil, garlic salt, pepper, salt, lime and juice to a bowl. Stir until combined.

Add the fish fillets, then rub the marinade all over them until they are completely covered.

Put it in the fridge for about an hour.

Now, place an aluminum foil sheet over a baking dish.

Place the fish over the top, then drizzle the marinade all over the fish.

As a parcel, fold the aluminum foil.

Bake it for around 30 to 40 minutes.

Allow it to cool.

Serve on a large plate with parsley sprinkled on top.

For extra flavor, you could drizzle some soya butter on top

These are just a few of the simple recipes that can be used to reduce stress and depress your mood. After going through the list of foods to combat stress and depression, you'll need to think of more. You can prepare some of them ahead of time and keep it in your fridge. You can reheat the dish and then eat it later.

# Conclusion

Through this book you will discover many methods for dealing with your depression. You will need to go back through the chapters and do the exercises again. This will make the exercises part of your daily routine.

If you can do this, it will help you to feel better about yourself. You will be more open to others and be able achieve your own level happiness.

You have the right to make your own decision. You can choose to become a statistic or you can respect yourself and work towards becoming less of a statistic. Depression can be caused by your thoughts becoming a source or allowing your surroundings to define you. By using the tips I have shared, you can get rid of depression and feel more healthy and happy.

www.ingramcontent.com/pod-product-compliance
Lightning Source LLC
Chambersburg PA
CBHW062116040426
42336CB00041B/1241